KV-281-798

Contents

Talking Health
Conventional and Complementary Approaches

Foreword by HRH The Prince of Wales

Edited by

Sir James Watt
Past President, Royal Society of Medicine

Associate Editor

Clive Wood
Linacre College, Oxford

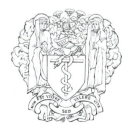

The Royal Society of Medicine

Royal Society of Medicine Services Limited
1 Wimpole Street London W1M 8AE
7 East 60th Street New York NY 10022

British Library Cataloguing in Publication Data

Talking health.
  1. Medicine
  I. Watt, J. (James), *1914–*
  II. Wood, Clive, *1940–*
  610

  ISBN 0-905958-64-0

Phototypeset by Dobbie Typesetting Ltd, Plymouth, Devon
Printed in Great Britain by Henry Ling Ltd, The Dorset Press, Dorchester, UK

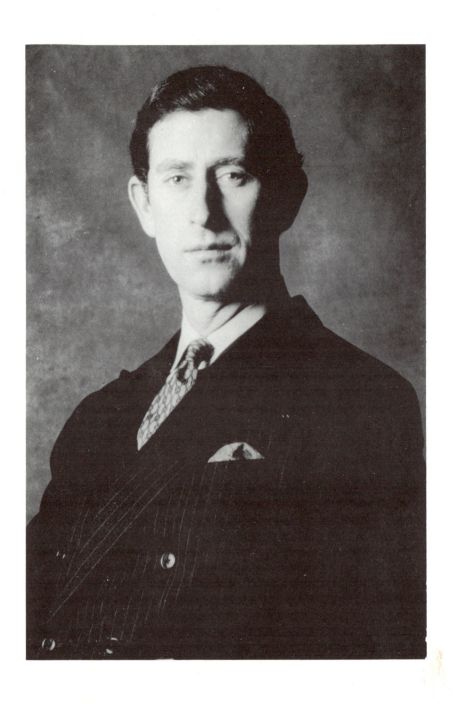

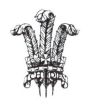

Having provoked a certain amount of discussion during the 150th anniversary of the British Medical Association, I was most encouraged when the Royal Society of Medicine decided to hold a series of Colloquia to debate what I consider to be a most important aspect of the *total* health care of individuals.

The Royal Society of Medicine has therefore rendered a valuable service to the future development of health care. Through hosting these Colloquia, your Society had given an opportunity, probably for the first time, for practitioners, both conventional and complementary, to come together to learn how each other think and work.

The importance of communication has been emphasised by all the practitioners who took part and it is particularly pleasing to observe how effective these Colloquia have been. Difficulties and differences are inevitable when dialogue of this nature is undertaken. The Colloquia on research and training are, I am sure, the preliminary exchanges in a much longer debate.

Scientific progress comes as much through deductive logic, rational debate and critical evaluation as it does through intuitive reasoning, creative play and the ability to tolerate uncertainty. The reports on the discussion indicate that both these essential strands to progress were maintained.

It has given me great pleasure to take part, albeit peripherally, in these Colloquia and I very much hope that, as a result of these gatherings, better ways will be found to deal with the myriad of problems that patients have. I also hope that, in the long run, a situation will develop by which the general practitioner can recommend genuine complementary therapists to treat his patients, if he feels that this is the more appropriate thing to do. I need hardly to say that I look forward to the continuation of the work that is so well described in this volume.

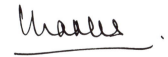

Preface

During Sir James Watt's Presidency from 1982 to 1984, the Royal Society of Medicine initiated a series of Colloquia on medicine and complementary therapies. Eight meetings were held between April 1984 and January 1987 under his chairmanship. They provided an opportunity for some members of the medical profession to discuss with practitioners of complementary therapies which have appropriate training, recognised qualifications and registration, what they could learn from each other that might be of public benefit.

The holding of these Colloquia demonstrates the Society's unique ability to provide a forum for the discussion of medical matters across all disciplines. From these meetings no Society view could emerge nor was it intended that it should, and the papers which follow solely represent the views of their authors.

I should like personally to acknowledge Sir James Watt's skilful guidance of the series and his commitment which contributed so greatly to the success of the Colloquia. I am also pleased to place on record the Society's gratitude to Lord Kindersley, whose support has been invaluable in the organisation and publication of these meetings.

Sir Gordon Robson,
President,
Royal Society of Medicine
1986–1988

Introduction:
An Attempt at Bridge Building

Sir James Watt
Past President, Royal Society of Medicine

In his address to the British Medical Association in 1983, the
Prince of Wales voiced his fear that our current preoccupation
with the sophistication of modern medicine would divert our
attention from "those ancient, unconscious forces, lying beneath
the surface, which still help to shape the psychological attitudes
of modern man". With his customary insight, His Royal
Highness was identifying a contemporary reaction against the
scientific determinism which, in the name of progress, has been
said to make us the prisoners of our own advances.

Prince Charles went on to suggest that "the whole imposing
edifice of modern medicine, for all its breathtaking successes is,
like the celebrated Tower of Pisa, slightly off balance". While
recognising the importance of maintaining and improving
professional standards, he believed that the art of healing should
nevertheless take account of the long-neglected complementary
therapies which, "in the right hands, can bring considerable
relief, if not hope to an increasing number of people."[1]

The French surgeon, biologist, and Nobel prize-winner,
Alexis Carrel, pointed out in 1935, that "man is an indivisible
whole of extreme complexity" who is not only the complex of
parts which might be analysed by scientific techniques, but who
is also an unknowable personality with a spiritual consciousness
that depends upon the integrity of the organism as a whole.

The error of the French philosopher Descartes, in Carrel's view,
had been to separate the mind from the body and to concentrate
the attention of doctors on organic disease. As he saw it, the
role of the doctor was to rescue the patient from the intellectual,
moral and physiological atrophy caused by contemporary life-
styles and restore him to health, which he defined as a well
integrated whole of intellectual, moral and organic activities in

1

a state of equilibrium. He pointed out that doctors, in fact, were more concerned with prevention, detection and treatment of organic disease and were less sensitive to the intellectual and moral conflicts which undermine spiritual health.[2]

Has much changed in this respect over the past 50 years since Carrel's day? Certainly, the research-based scientific advances have been spectacular and have brought relief, healing and often health to countless numbers of patients. The growth of knowledge has been such that specialties have had to develop, each competing for and making legitimate demands on the National Health Service budget which always falls short of the personnel and materials needed to benefit all those patients who are perceived by conventional methods of diagnosis to be ill. However, it has been estimated that one third of patients with chronic symptoms have no organic disease and that another third exhibit symptoms unrelated to their organic condition.[3] For them, for the understanding and for the relief of their suffering, the shortfall in expertise, funding (and time) is immense. Conventional medicine is unable to meet the needs of every patient.

Furthermore, in the tightly packed undergraduate curriculum with its emphasis on conventional teaching, practice and research, there seems as yet no prospect of amelioration of the situation so as to allow attention to be paid by the doctors of the future to those aspects of health alluded to by Alexis Carrel.

Again, the emphasis on research and technological development in hospital medicine and the pressure it exerts on those trained and training to high standards sometimes results in a patient becoming the impersonalised object of a battery of tests not necessarily related to his condition. This impersonalisation has extended to the moment of dying, and Fletcher has expressed the layman's concern about heroic attempts to resuscitate the terminally ill which deprive friends and relatives of "the classical death scene, with its loving partings and solemn words".[4] Society's growing determination to provide a caring environment and maintain human dignity in illness to the point of death is being witnessed in the steady growth of the hospice movement, though this voluntary effort goes only a small way to provide what is needed by all.

2

Holistic communication between patient and practitioner

Scientific advance and the intrusion of the machine have also, to some extent, affected the patient–doctor relationship to cause difficulties in communication. As Professor Margaret Turner-Warwick has observed: "Understanding between patient and doctor, that singularly personal relationship involving a complex mixture of often unfamiliar factors, emotions, hopes, fears and taboos, is continually confused by lay misconceptions, none of which may be declared but may, nevertheless, be deeply felt".[5] Such misconceptions may be why help is therefore sought from practitioners of complementary medicine, where patients can at least be assured of a listening ear, despite the fact that the majority declare themselves satisfied with the National Health Service. The complementary therapist has in general more time to talk and enquire into environmental factors which some overburdened doctors may overlook or regard as unimportant. The therapy offered usually involves the active participation of the patient, and this has obvious appeal in an age when authoritarianism, including that of the medical profession, is being challenged and health is considered to lie in self-help. The emergence of the College of Health with its emphasis upon this aspect of health promotion is indicative of this trend.

This is not to suggest that complementary practitioners are more "holistic" than orthodox medical practitioners, for the growing influence of the British Holistic Medical Association is evidence of the importance which many conventional doctors attach to the "whole person" approach. In fact, the integration of technological and scientific benefits with the development or re-creation of the patient's own self-healing and self-organising abilities can be accomplished in the highly specialised environment of the teaching hospital by teams of doctors, counsellors and therapists.[6,7]

Team work of this nature, which coordinates the many diverse factors involved in the healing process, was no doubt an objective which Prince Charles had in mind.

Responding to the challenge

The British Medical Association set up a Working Party under the auspices of its Board of Science and Education with a remit

3

"to consider the feasibility and possible methods of assessing the value of alternative therapies." The response of the Royal Society of Medicine was different. The original 1805 statutes of the Society allow it wide powers of discretion, for they state that: "The business of the Society . . . shall be to converse upon professional subjects and to read and hear Letters, Reports, and other papers on Medicine and in all its branches". The Society discharges this obligation through the meetings of its 33 Sections, representing most branches of medicine and surgery, through its interdisciplinary Forums on current socio-medical problems and through International Conferences. It has also a Section of Medical and Dental Hypnosis and an Open Section of lay members representing the public interest, who debate contemporary medical and ethical issues.

The Society was therefore admirably equipped to initiate a series of Colloquia on Conventional Medicine and Complementary Therapies which provide an opportunity for debate between members of relevant sections of the Society and professionally qualified complementary practitioners. Society members included a journalist, an historian, a pharmacist, a medical hypnotist and an Anglican priest engaged in the Church's healing ministry.

Because of the unsubstantiated claims made for a bewildering number of therapies by unqualified practitioners, we considered that meaningful discussion could only take place if all participants had been subjected to the discipline of academic study. We therefore invited only those complementary practitioners who met what we considered to be adequate professional criteria: comprehensive training, a recognized qualification and, allowing for the need to design appropriate research methodology, a willingness to submit their practice to the scientific rigour demanded of conventional medicine. Finally, they should have a desire to work towards the establishment of a register and possible regulatory body.

In the event, representatives of six therapies: osteopathy, chiropractic, acupuncture, homoeopathy, naturopathy and medical herbalism, agreed to take part in the Colloquia. They were matched by representatives from various relevant sections of the Royal Society of Medicine. We were able to proceed in a friendly and frank manner to compare and contrast our

4

respective philosophical and scientific concepts and our clinical management. We examined the problems encountered in designing suitable research protocols for therapies which were so diverse in character. We considered the advantages to the therapies of coordinating professional interests through a representative body responsible for a general register of complementary practitioners trained to an agreed standard. We were also able to compare our experience in the United Kingdom with that of other countries where public demand had led to similar inquiry.

Eight Colloquia: increasing dialogue

There were eight Colloquia in all, three of which were honoured by the presence of the Prince of Wales. Summaries of the papers and a synopsis of the main points made during the discussion periods appear in the body of the Report. The first of the Series was mainly exploratory and an attempt to break down barriers. It included an appeal by Dr Richard Tonkin for a constructive approach to collaboration in the light of growing public demand for complementary therapies, inadequate medical resources and the need to protect the public from charlatans. At this stage, however, it became evident that mutual distrust was responsible for the misgivings voiced by both conventional and complementary practitioners and would have to be overcome before identifying the problems and benefits of sharing their respective skills in the interest of the patient.

A step in that direction was provided, at the second Colloquium, by Dr Patrick Pietroni who showed how new scientific concepts had begun to cast doubt upon modern biomedical thinking. He questioned whether the scientific method, with its known limitations, could continue to be regarded as the only test of the appropriateness of therapy for human beings with their complex make-up, unique individuality and variable needs and responses. At the same time, he criticised the reluctance of complementary therapists to validate their healing methods and considered their training programmes as deficient in the humanitarian aspects of patient care as are the curricula of our medical schools.

The two Colloquia which followed provided practical comparisons of conventional and complementary approaches to clinical problems using video demonstrations of history-taking and examination of the patient. They displayed the professional attitude of the complementary practitioners which was something of a revelation to the orthodox practitioners present, although the discussion was somewhat inhibited and radical differences between orthodox and complementary approaches were not explored. The fifth Colloquium was therefore structured differently to allow more candid discussion in small groups on questions arising from a wide-ranging paper by Dr George Lewith on concepts common both to conventional and complementary medicine, which indicated areas of collaboration which might be fruitful, particularly in the fields of medical training, patient care and research. In his closing address, Professor Michael Baum, while paying tribute to the valuable lessons he had learnt from the Colloquia, was nevertheless at pains to stress the difference between science and non-science, the importance of validating therapy and the danger of both doctors and therapists intruding into the realm of spiritual healing, which was the proper province of the Church.

By the time of the sixth Colloquium, it had become apparent that complementary therapists recognised that they must be as willing as the doctors to engage in research to justify their practice. The climate of understanding, fostered by the Colloquia, made constructive discussion possible. Professor Ulrich Tröhler introduced the subject by showing how long it had taken medical scientists to evolve adequate research methodology and, after 400 years, it was still being refined. Dr Richard Tonkin, President of the Research Council for Complementary Medicine, explained some of the difficulties of conducting research in the complementary field, which included lack of manpower and resources, inadequate literature access and the need to modify research methodologies relevant to each therapy. However, he was also able to present the evidence of the Council's success in meeting the challenge.

The Colloquium was concluded with a review by Professor Ian McColl on the strengths and failures of both scientific medicine and complementary therapies, with examples of collaboration which worked for the well-being of the patient. He nevertheless challenged the therapists to face the implications of research, and described the improvements in surgical care at Guy's Hospital which had followed the weekly medical audit. Lack of facilities for research should not be considered a problem, because academic departments could offer the opportunity for complementary therapists to engage in mutually beneficial joint projects.

Is there need for legislation?
At this point in the Colloquia, it was clear that standards of training and practice, registration and regulation of therapies would influence the Government's attitude to future legislation. Baroness Trumpington, then Parliamentary Under Secretary of State in the Department of Health and Social Security, was therefore invited to address the seventh Colloquium on the Government's attitude towards conventional and complementary medicine. This, she suggested, was to reconcile freedom of choice with consumer protection, allowing the patient to seek the benefits of alternative medicines and therapies while, at the same time, ensuring that they were safe. All medicines, both conventional and alternative, would be subject to tests and, while she foresaw fewer problems for herbal remedies, the difficulties of assessing homoeopathic medicines might well prove insurmountable. The urgent need for research was thus reinforced. Finally, Baroness Trumpington emphasised the importance of therapists speaking with one voice if their desire for official recognition was to be gratified.

Sir David Innes Williams did not share the general optimism which had been generated by the Colloquia and warned of the opposition likely to be encountered from the medical profession if all practitioners were competing for the care of the same patient. He indicated some of the hurdles to be cleared and believed that a prime objective must be to reassure the medical profession.

The awakening of interest in what complementary therapies have to offer is a world-wide phenomenon and other governments have been obliged, because of public demand, to investigate their claims or to introduce legislation. There has been an Australian government inquiry and, in France, the efficacy of acupuncture and the manipulative therapies has been acccepted, while President Mitterand has called together a group

7

of scientists and complementary therapists to establish suitable methodologies for evaluating non-orthodox practices.[8]

It therefore seemed appropriate to consider, at the eighth and final Colloquium, patterns of collaboration in other countries. Professor J. C. van Es of the Department of General Practice at the Free University of Amsterdam described the situation in Holland. Dr Harold Gaier related the steps which led to the formation of the Associated Health Service Professions, of which he was Chairman, in South Africa and Mr Robert Duggan, Chairman of the Traditional Acupuncture Institute in Columbia, Maryland, discussed the changing scene in the United States with its implications for the future of medicine there.

As in the United Kingdom, features common to all three countries were increasing public demand, the distinction between qualified and unqualified therapists and a perception that agreed standards of training, research and registration under the aegis of a regulatory body was an essential prerequisite to official recognition and professional status.

In the United States, progress to this end was inhibited by the differing health regulations of 50 State Legislatures. Holland had bowed to public pressure by setting up a Commission for Alternative Systems of Medicine which had reported in 1981. It upheld the patient's right to choose, and made far-reaching recommendations which have not yet been adopted because of conflicting professional interests. The South African Government, on the other hand, showed surprising flexibility by creating an Associated Health Services Board which quickly established a model code of ethics and a six-year training course comparable to the medical student's curriculum.

The BMA Report

In the United Kingdom the report of the British Medical Association's Board of Science and Education on Alternative Therapy was published in May 1986.[9] As Baroness Trumpington points out, the report was helpful in identifying the sort of patient who might seek help from complementary therapists as distinct from the patient who needs the impressive resources which orthodox medicine has made available.

8

The main objective of the Report appears to have been to contrast the benefits brought by orthodox medicine through the application of the scientific method with the uncertain response believed to result from unproven therapies. Such therapies were described as deriving from discredited philosophies which were halting intellectual progress. The Working Party therefore found ''no logical class of alternative therapies: only therapies with and without good evidence for their efficacy''. Since evidence of efficacy, it was believed, could be provided by one or other form of scientifically controlled clinical trial, the technical and statistical aspects of such trials were explained in the report. Ethical aspects were not discussed, but Campbell has asked whether it can be morally right to withdraw therapy from patients who are benefitting from it or, as this form of trial demands, to deceive others.[10]

The BMA Working Party drew its evidence from a very wide spectrum of practitioners of alternative therapies. The Colloquia on the other hand dealt only with those professional bodies which met the Society's criteria. The Colloquia have shown that it is by no means as easy as the Working Party suggests to devise appropriate research protocols to validate complementary therapies. The way forward may depend on new scientific thinking already challenging the old orthodoxy.

The Commission for Alternative Systems of Medicine set up by the Netherlands Ministry of Health and Environmental Protection representing medical, paramedical and sociological disciplines, produced its report in 1981. The Commission believed that the division between orthodox and alternative systems of medicine was not primarily scientific but had its origin in political and social, as much as in scientific factors. It upheld the patient's right to choose between orthodox and complementary therapy and believed that controlled clinical trials of alternative therapies were impractical. The Commission made 11 recommendations which reflected many of the proposals made during the Colloquia.

The British Holistic Medical Association has published a detailed critique of the BMA Report which should be read in conjunction with it.[11]

9

The Church and lay person

When we came to review the material from the Colloquia, we became aware that it was deficient in two important respects. It lacked discussion on the role of spiritual healing, and informed comment on the attitudes of the public.

We are therefore grateful to the Reverend Christopher Hamel-Cooke, Rector of St Marylebone Parish Church with its Healing and Counselling Centre, who is a member of the Open Section of the Society and contributed actively to the Colloquia, for permission to reprint the chapter on Christian Counselling from his book *Health is for God*. Miss Katharine Whitehorn, columnist of the Observer, a past-president of the Open Section and staunch supporter of the Colloquia, has also been kind enough to contribute a *Layperson's View*, which reflects some of the confusion in the public mind to which Professor Turner-Warwick has drawn attention. Both contributions appear towards the end of this Report immediately before the concluding section on *Perceptions and Prospects*.

Acknowledgements

The programme and arrangements for each Colloquium were the responsibility of a small Planning Group, and it is a pleasure to acknowledge the valuable contributions of its members. The President and Council of the Royal Society of Medicine kindly provided the meeting facilities and Dr Graham Bennette, its Medical Services Secretary, willingly shouldered the immense administrative load, including the detailed minutes of each Colloquium on which this Report is based. He also played an essential coordinating role. Professor A. J. Harding Rains, Editor of the *Journal of the Royal Society of Medicine* has painstakingly reviewed the material and offered much helpful advice and criticism. Mr Robert Thomson, the Society's Executive Director, and Mr Howard Croft, its Director of Publications, have provided much practical assistance. Sir John Walton, Immediate Past President of the Royal Society of Medicine, took a close personal interest in the Colloquia and made many helpful observations.

We are also deeply grateful to Lord Kindersley for his staunch and generous support and for many constructive proposals.

Our greatest debt, however, is to His Royal Highness the Prince of Wales, without whose vision and stimulus this unique debate would never have occurred.

References

1 HRH The Prince of Wales. Presidential Address to the British Medical Association, 14 December 1982.
2 Carrel A. *Man the Unknown*. London: Hamish Hamilton 1936; 17, 118, 137, 140, 263, 273.
3 Weiss E, English O S. *Psychosomatic Medicine*. Third edition, Philadelphia: W B Saunders 1957; 4–5.
4 Fletcher J. *Moral Responsibility: Situation Ethics at Work*. London: SCM Press, 1967; 147.
5 Turner-Warwick M. The problem of misunderstanding the misunderstood. *The Times* 1975, June 15.
6 Nixon P G F. Stress, life style and cardiovascular disease. A cardiological odyssey. *British Journal of Holistic Medicine* 1984; 1: 20–9.
7 Pinney S, Freeman L J, Nixon P G F. Role of the nurse counsellor in managing patients with the hyperventilation syndrome. *Journal of the Royal Society of Medicine*, 1987; **80**: 216–8.
8 Editorial. Le président et les thérapies non-conventionnelles. *Le Monde* 1985, March 6: p. 12.
9 British Medical Association Report of the Board of Science and Education on Alternative Therapy. London: BMA, 1986.
10 Campbell A V. *Moral Dilemmas in Medicine*. Edinburgh: Churchill Livingstone, 1982: 72.
11 British Holistic Medical Association. Report on the BMA Board of Science Working Party on Alternative Therapy. London: BHMA, 1986.

11

Comparisons and Contrasts

Both conventional and complementary practitioners agree that the needs of the patient are paramount, but their approach to these needs is governed by radically different concepts. Whilst all good practitioners approach their patient "holistically", these two healing traditions differ, both in philosophy and in practice. Patients may perceive that the complementary therapist is perhaps able to give them greater time and more detailed, personal attention, while the orthodox practitioner has a greater therapeutic armamentarium to offer.

In this Section, George Lewith describes the different approaches to illness taken by therapists from different traditions. Ian McColl calls on orthodox medicine to put its own house in order and Michael Baum makes a plea that we should start to distinguish science from faith. Both have their place in healing and the art of medicine is to identify and meet the patient's individual need.

Common Concepts in Conventional and Complementary Medicine

George T Lewith
Centre for the Study of Alternative Therapies, Southampton, SO1 2DG, UK

As clinicians there is one thing that we can all agree on: to all of us in a clinical setting, *the patient comes first*. Our main aim as clinicians is to define the best and most appropriate treatment for any individual, taking into account their physical illness along with its social, emotional and spiritual components.

Increasing interest in complementary therapies

Perhaps therefore, the first question to ask is why growing numbers of people are seeking treatment with complementary therapies. We recently surveyed all the new patients attending our clinic in Southampton, over a period of one month. Sixty-five patients were seen at the initial interview and 56 of these were followed up some two months later. Although 20% of the clinic time is spent seeing patients who are socially disadvantaged either free of charge or for a nominal fee, the largest group of patients attending the Centre were in Social Class II, married and female, aged between 26 and 50.[1]

Patients came with a variety of problems, most of which had been present for a long time. Only three patients had been referred to the Centre by medical colleagues. The vast majority stated that failure of conventional medicine was their main reason for seeking complementary therapies, although they had a good relationship with their general practitioner and felt that they had received satisfactory treatment through the National Health Service. Patients interviewed after the first consultation felt that the complementary therapist understood their problems and could, as a consequence, provide a successful and effective form of therapy.

We felt that these patients were not cranks and had not lost confidence or interest in conventional medicine, but were seeking

15

a solution to an unresolved long-term problem. Our study showed that approximately 60% of patients attending the Centre felt much better after therapy. An important reason for the apparent satisfaction, and clinical success of complementary therapies, in this study, may have something to do with the therapies themselves. If this is correct, then the concepts underpinning these therapies deserve close examination as they may have a valuable contribution to make to our understanding of some illnesses.

Doctors, particularly those in general practice, are also becoming far more interested in complementary therapies. A recent limited study from the Institute of Complementary Medicine, published in September 1984, suggested an increase of 20% in the provision of complementary therapies by non-medically trained practitioners between mid-1983 and mid-1984.

A survey completed this year by a Bath general practitioner, Dr Richard Wharton and myself, funded by the Research Council for Complementary Medicine, looked at the attitude of a random sample of 195 general practitioners in the Avon region to complementary therapies. Over half perceived these therapies as either useful or very useful and were regularly referring patients to complementary therapists. Approximately half of those referrals were to registered, but non-medically qualified, people.[2]

Thus, it would appear that a significant shift has already occurred in the attitudes of both patients and general practitioners, in their approach to this area of medicine. The recent BMA enquiry into complementary therapies seemed to be based on the tacit assumption that doctors could somehow investigate and, if necessary, veto these therapies if they considered them to be quackery. From the information we have available, such an attitude would appear to be misplaced; our attitudes should be much more open and realistic.

Models of illness

Certain models of illness, in both conventional and complementary medicine, reveal that areas of common ground are shared by these two approaches. Let us consider, for example, the condition of peptic ulcer, and examine the approach of a clinical ecologist, a homoeopath and a conventional doctor. All three clinicians would take a history from the patient. The clinical ecologist, or food allergist, would be particularly interested in any past history of illness, with particular reference to allergic symptoms such as asthma and eczema in childhood. He would also wish to take a very detailed history of the foods which might precipitate, aggravate or alleviate the abdominal pain and this history would form the basis upon which he would begin to select the foods that the patient must exclude from his diet. Most clinical ecologists are medically trained, and would probably refer the patient for investigations such as a barium meal or gastroscopy, if these had not already been done prior to the consultation.

The homoeopath may or may not be medically qualified. He would also consider the history in great detail, particular attention being paid to the description of pain, its location and its radiation. He would consider a range of factors that might aggravate or alleviate the pain, such as food, ambient temperature or the patient's emotional state. The classical Kentian homoeopath would then attempt to arrive at the appropriate single homoeopathic remedy which will allow effective treatment of the ulcer.

The conventional doctor would consider the factors that aggravate and alleviate the abdominal pain and the history would certainly be shorter than that taken by the clinical ecologist or the homoeopath. All three practitioners would examine the patient's abdomen to be sure that there were no masses or other significant clinical findings.

The illness model in the mind of each of these three practitioners also differs. The conventional doctor views ulcers as being caused by the breakdown of the gastro–intestinal tract's normal competence, due to factors such as the over-production of gastric acid, or emotional stress. The clinical ecologist views the development of gastro–intestinal disease as resulting from the body's failure to deal with the physical stresses imposed on it by a food to which it is intolerant. This idea of food *intolerance* rather than food *allergy* seems a much more appropriate concept to describe the ecologist's approach, and one that is less likely to be challenged by those who are immunologically trained.

17

The homoeopath may believe that the patient's genetic constitution predisposes to the development of ulcers, or that the ulcer may be caused by some insult to the liver that disturbs its energetic function. Such energetic dysfunction would not result in abnormal liver enzymes, but would be thought to result from a pathological process occurring in the stomach or duodenum.

Each practitioner will be looking for slightly different clues. The complementary practitioner would probably take a more thorough history than the conventional doctor and might therefore be better able to isolate the environmental and psychological elements aggravating or causing the ulcer. Conventional medicine may be guilty of imposing its own illness model on patients and the doctor may therefore fail to understand patients' needs, and as a consequence fail to help them.

The detailed investigative techniques that could be used by the conventional doctor would, assuming that the ulcer was benign, probably lead to a single therapy, whatever the cause of the ulcer. This might be the use of cimetidene or a similar drug to reduce the gastric acid and allow the ulcer to heal. The complementary practitioner would have at his disposal less sophisticated investigations, but would be using a much broader approach to therapy. If he believed the ulcer was caused by emotional pressure then he would be more likely to recommend the appropriate psycho–therapeutic procedures designed to alleviate or control the patient's response.

Two types of illness

General practitioners, often unconsciously, tend to divide illness into two main groups. One presents with a constellation of symptoms and signs that indicate a specific diagnosis, such as a peptic ulcer, rheumatoid arthritis or a cerebrovascular accident. The other, more common, category is that of "undifferentiated" illness. Patients often present with a vague group of symptoms such as headache, malaise and abdominal distension. They are rarely, if ever, seen by hospital specialists, because they simply do not fit into a defined disease pattern. Detailed investigations in such patients are almost invariably normal and the general practitioner is often left with a patient who is unwell but cannot be given a firm diagnosis.[3]

The Royal College of General Practitioners has developed an excellent model for training GPs to deal with such illness. They consider the interrelated triad of its social, psychological and physical aspects. Such an approach requires a complete understanding of detailed family relationships and involves viewing the illness over a period of time in the context of its environment. This allows for the illness to be considered and managed by combining a range of primarily psychological and pharamaceutical approaches for particular patients and specific problems.

The clinical ecologist has a similar model for illness. A reaction to wheat may produce symptoms varying from an undiagnosable illness to a clearly defined migraine or an active and serologically positive rheumatoid arthritis. Furthermore, the symptoms produced by specific foods may change with time. An individual with milk intolerance may develop eczema as a small child, asthma at about the age of six and finally migraine in the mid twenties. All of these symptoms or diseases could potentially be resolved by avoiding milk. The clinical ecologist's approach does however take into account more than just simple food intolerance. If a patient who was previously stable and well controlled on a food exclusion diet suffers from considerable emotional stress, then the symptoms may return and sometimes new or more complex food intolerances develop. In other words, psychological pressures can have a clear and often reproduceable effect on clinically measurable disease.[4]

Both the clinical ecologist and the general practitioner therefore view undifferentiated illness as a complex problem in which physical, spiritual and psychological stressors play an interrelated and often changeable role in the development and natural history of the condition. A detailed understanding of complementary medicine may allow the conventional practitioner to develop a much more accurate understanding of the cause of a particular illness, and, as a consequence, a much better grasp of its treatment. The complementary practitioner, who does not have a formal medical training, would also benefit from a more detailed understanding of conventional medicine as this would add substantially to both his understanding of illness and his diagnostic abilities.

Biological energy

One of the main ideas that underpin all complementary therapies is that of biological energy, which in the case of traditional Chinese medicine is termed *chi*. The homoeopath, osteopath, naturopath and acupuncturist all view the manipulation of this indefinable vital force as the essential factor in successful therapy. All primitive, and by implication intuitive, medical systems have had some idea of vital force as the basis of their medical systems. Conventional medicine does not have such concepts and therefore finds difficulty in defining health.

However, the traditional Chinese view of illness cannot be sustained as a theory if it fails to produce adequate results in the context of clinical practice. Therefore some attempt must be made to analyse the philosophy of traditional Chinese medicine in terms of treatment outcome. Such research, particularly in the field of acupuncture, has unfortunately been bedevilled by a number of misunderstandings. All too often, conventional doctors have seen acupuncture purely as a stimulation technique that involves the insertion of needles in or around a site of pain. Research protocols designed to evaluate complementary therapies must take into account their whole philosophy. This lack of understanding has led to many inadequate research projects and made comparisons between different therapeutic approaches difficult if not impossible.

Modern pharmacology is firmly rooted in conventional reductionist views and as a consequence finds it very difficult to understand the underlying principle of homoeopathy, based as it is on the assumption that infinitesimal doses of a substance may have a dramatic effect. However, there are reports that rats given a dose of carbon tetrachloride that would normally cause severe liver damage and death, can be protected by the prior administration of 15C potency of carbon tetrachloride which does not contain any material strength, and therefore when analysed would simply be pure water. The effects of a dose of copper which would normally stunt and destroy the growth of wheat seedlings can apparently also be overcome by preloading the seedlings with a 15C potency of copper. Such experiments suggest that there may be more to homoeopathy than our logical approach to pharmacology may at first allow us to accept.[5]

Towards a broader view of "science"

Although therapeutic fashions change, the ideas underlying our approach to illness tend to remain consistent. There are many strong conceptual similarities between conventional and complementary medicine, but there is a need for new thinking if conventional medicine is to progress. The complex nature of the body's response to acupuncture and the therapeutic conundrums of homoeopathy may represent fundamental truths through which we can find new ways of looking at illness and its treatment. However, without adequate support and research funding, the complementary therapist will continue to be outmanoeuvred academically and this may ultimately mean that patients are denied potentially valuable treatments. Science, in the literal sense, means knowledge. The so-called scientific reductionist approach held up by many conventional doctors as "pure science", (eg. measurement) is simply one interpretation of the way of acquiring knowledge. "Science" (knowledge) by measurement, must not be used as an academic truncheon. We must approach these issues with an open mind.

References
1 Moore J, Phipps K, Marcer D, Lewith G. Why do people seek treatment by alternative medicine? *British Medical Journal* 1985; **290**: 28–9.
2 Wharton R, Lewith G. Complementary medicine and the general practitioner, *British Medical Journal* 1986; **292**: 1498–1500.
3 Lewith G, ed. *Alternative Therapies*. London: Heinemann, 1985.
4 Lewith G, Kenyon J. *Clinical Ecology*. Wellingborough: Thorsons, 1985.
5 Kenyon J. *Modern Techniques of Acupuncture* Volume 2. Wellingborough: Thorsons, 1983: 13–42.

Can Orthodox and Complementary Medicine Come Together?

Ian McColl

Department of Surgery, Guy's Hospital, London, SE1 9RT, UK

The medical profession does not view complementary medicine with any real hostility. Many of us have been impressed by orthopaedic surgeons having their own backache treated by osteopaths and we have listened with interest to pharmacologists stressing that homoeopathic drugs do no harm in contrast to many orthodox medicines. As a youngster I was impressed by the quiet, charming and unpatronising manner of our homoeopathic doctor.

The increasing public interest in complementary medicine may in part be due to the feeling that orthodox medicine often pays inadequate attention to the patient as a whole. For instance, a family doctor took her son with a broken arm to a surgeon and the treatment was completely successful. On none of the three occasions that the mother took her son to the clinic did the surgeon look or speak to her or to her son; he only examined the arm. Not a single word to either of them did he ever utter.

The lack of time is often blamed for these deficiencies with orthodox medicine and there is no doubt that complementary medical practitioners do have more time to spend with their patients. Nevertheless, the overriding deficiency is often seen as one of attitude. We would do well to heed what the patients say. The patient is the customer and the customer is always right.

Need for clinical trials

We have acknowledged the need for controlled clinical trials to validate complementary therapies and also a good deal of conventional medicine. Most prove difficult to reach a conclusion, however well designed the trials may be. It was interesting that a recent trial on the treatment of backache showed no statistical difference between physiotherapy and osteopathy.

There is naturally some concern about those therapies which are disruptive to the patient, his way of life, and the life of his family. Take for instance the man of 70 dying of inoperable cancer of the brain. A good neurologist explains to him kindly and gently what the prognosis is. The patient chooses an alternative therapy which unfortunately involves an unpleasant dietary regime whose advocates deny him his usual evening glass of whisky and the steak which he has enjoyed for so long. He is put on an appalling diet, the preparation of which occupies half the household for most of the day. Therapies that produce this kind of deprivation and disruption are naturally regarded with considerable suspicion.

In a later chapter, Dr Tonkin remarks that there are many factors involved in treating patients, several of them important but impossible to control, and I am reminded of a general practitioner in South East London, treating a young girl with pneumonia before the War. He was a very good family doctor and suggested to the father that a second opinion should be sought just to make sure that he was taking the right course of action. He called in a physician from the local hospital who elicited a careful history and did a thorough examination. He confirmed that all was being done that could be done. He collected a small fee and went home in his small car.

The father was not impressed by this. He wanted something much better. So the wise family doctor called in a different sort of consultant, whose name might have been Sir Trumpington Appleby. He arrived in morning dress in his chauffeur-driven Rolls Royce. He swept into the house taking little time with the history or the examination and summoned the whole family. The situation, he said, was very grave indeed and they must all work together. He gave them all jobs to do—"You will clean the windows every half hour"; "you will wash the floor every two hours"; "you will open the window for five minutes every half hour" and so on. After collecting a large fee he swept out and off in his Rolls Royce. They were all very impressed indeed. Some patients may be benefitted by such a swash-buckling performance with its large fee and occupational therapy. It is difficult to control these immeasurable factors, but we cannot deny that they play a role.

Checking the claims

What about unusual claims? I think it would be very helpful to have some of the more unusual practices examined, as I am sure they are being studied by the Research Council for Complementary Medicine. Perhaps they would look at page 7 of the British Chiropractic Handbook, which says that chiropractors may treat a small number of visceral complaints that are known by experience to respond to such treatment. Clinical and spinal subluxations are said to cause neurophysiological defects in the autonomic nervous system, and manipulation may cure problems like vertigo and bronchial asthma, catarrh and indigestion.

Forms of collaboration

In a surgical field hospital on the Thai–Campuchea border, traditional healers are prepared to supply alternative treatments to those who want them. The therapists chew a variety of herbal concoctions and then spit on the bandaged wounds of those who wish to have such therapy. They also give large quantities of herbal preparations, up to 1–2 litres a day, which helps restore the fluid balance. These herbs have a pleasant smell and the European doctors have them spit on their infected mosquito bites, which apparently affords them relief. In the evenings they give steam baths and massage both to the patients and the doctors. This illustrates an important principle. The two groups of therapists are working together and the local patients are happy with the arrangement.

Looking to the future, Dr Patrick Pietroni suggests that complementary practitioners should work in some well chosen general practice or health centres, so that a mutual language can be developed and sensible trials planned.

Another advantage of the general practice environment involving complementary therapists is that more attention could be given to self-help. There is very good evidence that if we help our patients to create a more peaceful state of mind within themselves, their whole well-being will be improved. The general practice environment, with complementary therapists present, would provide a good atmosphere for practising truly holistic medicine, for giving the patient a greater say about what sort

25

of treatment he wants. Of course, not everyone wants to have holistic medicine. Some prefer to be given drugs to suppress their symptoms. They do not want people prying into their personal affairs, uncovering the facts which they would prefer to remain hidden. Many problems might be more easily unravelled with this arrangement.

A distinguished physician with an international reputation was once asked by the parents of a child who was very ill indeed "Would you mind, doctor, if we took her to Lourdes? It would be no reflection on your treatment, but we would like to take her there". He replied "No, I certainly have no objection. We are going to need all the help we can get".

We all need to keep an open mind in the interests of the patients we serve. Humility has never claimed a monopoly of truth.

Science versus Non-science in Medicine: Fact or Fiction*

Michael Baum

Department of Surgery, King's College School of Medicine and Dentistry, London SE5 9LU, UK

"Don't underestimate the importance of an awareness of what lies beneath the surface of the visible world and of those ancient unconscious forces which still help to shape the psychological attitudes of modern man. Sophistication is only skin deep and when it comes to healing people it seems to me that account has to be taken of those sometimes long-neglected complementary methods of medicine".

The above quotation comes from the address made by HRH Prince Charles to the British Medical Association to mark its 150th anniversary. It is appropriate therefore to acknowledge from the start the efforts of the Prince which have been the catalyst in establishing a dialogue between the disparate membership of the Royal Society of Medicine's Colloquia on Conventional Medicine and Complementary Therapies.

Nevertheless, there have been occasions during the early meetings of this group when a robust and healthy argument has been forfeited for an exchange of generalities couched in the language of polite diplomacy. For example, if I would stand up at a meeting of the Royal Geological Society and claim that the earth was flat, there would no doubt be members of the audience who would leap to their feet to refute such a suggestion. I am sure that vigorous debate would have been welcomed, and enjoyed, but in the event, those present during the first two or three Colloquia seem to have been inhibited. My personal explanation for the cause of such inhibition is that none of us wish to see ourselves portrayed as reactionary stereotypes. In particular, members of the orthodox medical profession fear to have

---

* Reprinted with kind permission from the *Journal of the Royal Society of Medicine* 1987; 80: 332–3.

themselves exposed as establishment figures with closed minds and a lack of compassion. Yet I am sure that on a number of occasions during the earlier Colloquia we have felt like the little boy in Hans Christian Andersen's tale of the *Emperor's New Clothes*.

Failings of conventional medicine

Nonetheless I learnt a number of very valuable lessons from attending these meetings, and I recognize that in conventional medicine we certainly have at least two failings. We frequently fail as communicators with our patients and we frequently fail to fulfil the pastoral role that our clients require of us. But in our defence it is difficult to know just to what extent it is appropriate for a doctor to assume a pastoral role. I think it is presumptuous for us to encroach in a flat-footed and unskilled way into the territory of the clergy, but I have no doubt at all that any good doctor, trained within any of our medical schools, should approach his work with patients in a holistic manner. It seems to me that many complementary therapists, and others interested in these approaches, have hijacked the idea of holism. It is true, of course, that there are doctors who are not very good at their job, who do not handle their patients and their illness in a holistic manner. Doubtless the same is true of complementary therapists, but it must be refuted as sheer nonsense to say that conventional medicine is not holistic in its outlook.

In both the biological and psychological spheres and at their interface, contemporary research and clinical investigations are holistic. It is nonsensical to expect a rigid Cartesian model of a human being to give any kind of satisfactory account of the phenomena of homoeostasis, yet there are subtle differences between the types of holism which we practise and that which fringe practitioners preach. The ideas of holism described by our complementary colleagues are completely metaphysical and relate to some as yet undiscovered, and for all we know non-existent, ''natural life force'', whereas in orthodox medicine our concepts of holism are based on well defined neuroendocrine pathways which are known to link the psyche and the soma. Furthermore, we can recognize, measure and manipulate the chemical and cellular messages that pass throughout the body linking cell to cell and organ to organ, which in health act in perfect concert.

Many homoeopathic practitioners choose to stigmatize drugs such as cimetidine as powerful allopathic repressive therapy that poisons the natural reparative capacity of the body. I choose to look upon this group of drugs as restoring the natural harmony between the sympathetic and para-sympathetic nervous systems, following which established mucosal ulcers will heal under the natural stimuli of local cellular growth factors and hormones. We *know* this class of drug will heal established ulcers, prevent bleeding and perforation and avoid the necessity for surgery. Homoeopathy, acupuncture and meditation have no such *proven* record, for all their efforts to restore the balance of hypothetical natural fluxes.

Returning once more to the pastoral role of the physician, let us consider the term "undifferentiated illness", a popular description for many patients consulting homoeopathists. I believe that alternative models exist to describe and explain this condition. For example, I may choose to describe undifferentiated illness as the somatic manifestation of unhappiness. Unhappiness may be a result of loss of faith or psychological trauma in our childhood or adolescence. Perhaps these unhappy people would be better off seeking the ministry of the Church, or consulting a psychotherapist. To describe the popular obsession with complementary medicine in the treatment of "undifferentiated illness" as a failure of orthodox medicine is therefore only one interpretation of the truth. Alternative explanations might invoke a failure of the Church to cope with contemporary social problems, or a disenchantment with the psychotherapeutic model in modern society. My own personal prejudice would be to classify "undifferentiated illness" as a spiritual malaise requiring an infusion of spiritual solace rather than exposure to the pseudo-scientific gobbledegook of the acupuncturist.

We all of us have our faiths, but to try and convert a Christian who should be seeking spiritual solace in his Church to a course of homoeopathy whenever he or she is unhappy, should be seen as an activity in the realm of proselytism.

Science and non-science

In order to clarify our thinking at this point, it is important that we make a clear distinction between what is science and what is non-science. For a start, non-science does not mean nonsense, but non-science has to be equated with the areas of faith that cannot be subjected to tests of validation or refutation. The characteristic feature of the scientific method which distinguishes it from the area of faith is that scientists are prepared to expose all their favoured hypotheses to the hazards of refutation. In other words, true scientists are intellectually honest. This does not mean that they lack imagination, because the first step in the scientific method involves the construction of a hypothesis which by its very nature is a creation of imaginative flair. It is always possible to corroborate your hypothesis by inductive reasoning, seeking only the evidence that supports your ideas and ignoring or blinding yourselves to any contradictory data. There will, of course, be examples in the history of science where great ideas have gained spectacular corroboration by use of the inductive process alone. For example, William Harvey described the circulation of the blood 100 years before Anthoni von Leeuwenhoek demonstrated the capillaries, following the invention of the microscope. Now in historical terms (using the retrospectroscope) we can say that Harvey's brilliant leap of imagination turned out to be one of the most important milestones in the development of medical science, yet it would be a dangerous syllogism to argue that any brilliant leap of imagination is an idea ahead of its time. So, for the day-to-day purposes of evaluating scientific claims we still require painstaking, laborious and above all honest deductive research. If it is stated to be impossible to design the scientific research protocols to test the validity of a therapeutic claim, then such claims must be judged to be within the realm of faith and valued accordingly.

The hazards of faith masquerading as science are to be experienced both within the realms of orthodox and complementary medicine. Where the treatments on offer are non-invasive and non-toxic, as is mostly the case in complementary medicine (and provided the patient is not denied truly effective therapy), there is no real danger. However, when the treatments on offer are mutilating and life-threatening, as may be the case in orthodox medicine, then the hazards of inductivism are self-evident. Happily there can be a high degree of congruence on methods of evaluation of therapy, and certainly there are many areas in complementary medicine that lend themselves to the conventional scientific method. At the same time, there are certain approaches that cannot be evaluated using the scientific paradigm, and assuming that patients are not denied proven remedies or subjected to dangerous abuses, we can rest content with the knowledge that such approaches are a substitute for faith.

Searching for a common language

Science and non-science share no common ground in our metaphysical approach to life but they certainly share common aims, which are to improve the quality as well as the length of an individual's life and at the end improve the quality of dying. Furthermore, what is non-science today may indeed become the science of tomorrow and with these thoughts in mind the complacencies of both schools of thought must be shaken. I recently addressed a conference at St Galen in Switzerland entitled *Krebs und Alternativa Medizina*. Mine was the only paper read in English and was therefore the only one I understood. For the rest of the day I suffered the frustration and boredom of sitting through a series of papers both from orthodox and complementary therapists without understanding the language.

In contrast, at these Colloquia we have begun to understand each other and we must use this fine start to the best advantage to accommodate the ideas and precepts of science and those of complementary therapies. We must look for a single standard of high quality research that will be applicable to both areas of investigation and we must continue to search for a language that all of us can understand. In the meantime, perhaps the best compromise between the apparently contradictory claims of mystery and the mind is to remember Bayne's dictum: "We have to see that the spirit must lean on science as its guide in the world of reality and that science must turn to the spirit for the meaning of life".

Comparisons and Contrasts
Highlights from the Discussions

No monopoly on holism

Lord Kindersley noted that the word "Colloquium" was first used in 1609 to signify "an assembly for discussion". It was most important that the work of the medical profession and the complementary therapists, which often overlapped, should be understood by the public. These Colloquia should go a long way towards fulfilling this aim.

Professor Baum pointed out that, despite what had been implied, orthodox practitioners did not particularly use Cartesian principles in their work. There were simply "good doctors" and "bad doctors". For example, great attention was currently being given by clinical oncologists to the question of psychosocial factors in cancer. A recent survey conducted by the Imperial Cancer Campaign had shown a relatively high level of confidence among members of the general public in the performance of the medical profession.

Dr Gilbertson agreed that the concept of holism should not be identified with any particular group, and in his speciality of anaesthetics and intensive care, there was a growing emphasis on the significance of psychosocial factors.

The Reverend Christopher Hamel-Cooke described the support that was being provided by clergy and doctors working side by side in his Parish of St Marylebone. Pressures of inner city living created a great need for this type of ministry which involved cooperation between the clergy, the medical profession, qualified complementary therapists and lay counsellors.

Mr Mills disclaimed any wish on the part of serious complementary therapists to monopolise the concept of holism. However, in the past 50 years, it had been increasingly recognised that some complementary approaches were of particular value in non-organic illness, if only because of their emphasis on restorative and regenerative stimulation of the

33

natural healing potential of the individual, rather than on intervention techniques.

Colonel Baraclough deplored the fact that there was little or no control of certain complementary practitioners, for example lay homoeopaths. It was imperative to introduce legislation in order to protect patients.

Lord Kindersley pointed out that the Colloquia involved only those practitioners associated with recognised professional qualifications. He acknowledged, however, the urgent need to find means of achieving common standards.

Mr Hutchinson said that collaboration with general practitioners would be much easier if a professional register existed. At present it was difficult for doctors to know to whom they ought to refer patients even for private treatment.

Mr Lambert considered that the involvement of complementary therapy in the National Health Service was desirable but could only be considered in principle at present, owing to the limited number of accredited and registered therapists available who would be swamped by the workload generated by any NHS commitment.

Mr Hutchinson believed that there was a danger of splitting healing and science into two separate, and even opposing, camps. Medicine was not exclusively a science. The art of medicine had long been acknowledged. A paper in the *Lancet*[1] suggested that patients who attended chiropractors developed a better awareness of their condition because they felt that they had a more equal relationship with the therapist. He was not defending the complementary approach as such, for all practitioners were essentially "complementary". But the art of medicine was lost if the importance of the doctor–patient relationship was overlooked.

Dr Fraser Steele found no need to question the immense value of science in treatment. The main task of the Colloquia was to ask practical questions that would lead to cooperation between the two groups. Accreditation was one obvious requirement. It was immensely important to present the accredited practice of both conventional and complementary therapies to the public in an orderly and intelligible way.

Mr Burn, as a surgeon, found himself frequently faced with life-threatening conditions. Here the necessities of the situation did not call for a philosophical assessment but for the practical need to arrive at the best possible diagnosis. It was his view that complementary therapy should only be available within the National Health Service if its efficacy could be demonstrated within that context.

Dr Tonkin noted that whatever the pros and cons of investigating the success of complementary therapies, the ever increasing number of patients with minimal, non-specific or chronic illness would mean that such therapists were increasingly consulted.

HRH The Prince of Wales, who attended the Fourth Colloquium, believed that a problem existed in choosing the right words in addressing such questions as, "What is science?" and "What is truth?". There were many definitions of the nature of science and the notion of truth was changing all the time. In medicine there was perhaps too little attention given to feeling and intuition. People worried that complementary therapies might be dismissed as nonsense by the experts, though they knew of countless instances where help had been provided. We must develop better sensitivity to each person as a unique individual with a spiritual fingerprint. The type of healing that may not work for one might work for someone else.

Approaching the patient as a person
The Third Colloquium compared, by means of video, the ways in which practitioners elicited various significant features in the history of a patient complaining of back pain. During the Fourth Colloquium, a film was shown of a medical herbalist, an acupuncturist and a consultant gastroenterologist examining the same patient, whose principal illness, a peptic ulcer, was related to problems of personality and life-style.

Sir James Watt summarised the main conclusions that had emerged from the video demonstrations during the two Colloquia and the discussions which had followed:-
1. Time was needed to discover the person. It was a lack of time that so often turned a patient into a "case" demanding a diagnostic label which identified the routine treatment that

was to be given. However, careful history-taking and examination had uncovered, in both instances, complex problems underlying the persisting symptoms.

2. The need for a properly structured interviewing technique had been demonstrated.

3. A holistic approach had to be sustained over the whole period of the encounter with the patient. Osteopaths and chiropractors had shown how new factors in the patient's history could be elicited during the course of a full physical examination which was used by them to promote relaxation and to strengthen the bond of confidence between the practitioner and the patient. Perhaps doctors had something to learn from this.

4. Nevertheless, the general practitioner had a unique opportunity of assisting the patient through continuing contact and good doctors modified their treatment in relation to their perceptions of the patient's changing needs. This was appreciated by many patients.

5. The complex nature of the illnesses of both patients revealed that there was often a need for therapeutic help from a team with diverse skills including counselling.

6. Sympathetic cooperation, based upon respect for professional competence and recognition of what each had to contribute was a realistic objective and should temper future discussions.

7. Such discussion, however, was likely to be inhibited for want of a common language, since each discipline used its own terms to describe its philosophies and techniques. Exponents of the various disciplines must therefore endeavour to clarify the terms they used if collaboration was to become meaningful.

An acceptable basis for collaboration

During the Fifth Colloquium, a discussion group addressed the question "What will provide an acceptable basis, for collaboration between the medical profession and the complementary therapists?".

Members of this panel felt that the experience of the Third World was valuable, where traditional and conventional medicine came together in a position of equality. They hoped that such equality could be achieved in the West. Indeed, without it any attempts at dialogue would fail. The discussion group had considered the role of the Council for Complementary and Alternative Medicine (CCAM), composed of the professional bodies representing acupuncture, chiropractic, osteopathy, homoeopathy, medical herbalism and naturopathy. The Council's main work was concerned with ethics, discipline and education. It was considered that training approved by the CCAM should reach the same standard as that of the basic medical sciences in orthodox medicine and that the clinical training of complementary practitioners should make them competent to decide when their treatment was appropriate to the patient's condition and when the patient should be referred to a medical practitioner. On the other hand, the medical profession should become more aware of what complementary therapies could do for their patients. It was desirable to eliminate the less commendable features of both orthodox and complementary practice. This might be achieved by seeing some patients together. Any attempt at dialogue would require the development of a common language since much specialist jargon was unintelligible to members of other disciplines.

In summary, it was felt that training in complementary medicine should be comparable to that in orthodox medicine because training held the key to future collaboration. More should be done to enable general practitioners to understand the principles and practice of complementary medicine. Comparable training and better insights should lead to mutual respect and confidence.

Reference

1 Kane R L, Leymaster C, Olsen D, Woolley F R, Fisher F D. Manipulating the patient: a comparison of the effectiveness of physician and chiropractor care. *Lancet* 1974; 1; 1333–6.

Directions for Research

It is generally believed, both by complementary and by orthodox practitioners, that research to "validate" complementary approaches would aid their more widespread acceptance. It is seldom realised that the research designs currently in use are of fairly recent origin. It is also becoming increasingly clear that such designs may not be the most appropriate for the study of complementary therapies. However, any newer approaches to evaluation are slow to gain acceptance. The whole question of research is therefore in something of a quandary.

Ulrich Tröhler charts the rise of statistically-based scientific research, starting in the Eighteenth Century but only being fully developed in the last 50 years.

Patrick Pietroni suggests that there are many ways of acquiring knowledge. The scientific method is only one, along with experience, insight and intuition. And we live in a universe of participation. To study man away from his environment is like looking at fish out of water.

Richard Tonkin considers that for several reasons complementary therapists will find research difficult to pursue. One solution, he suggests, is greater collaboration between orthodox practitioners, who are well used to scientific enquiry, and complementary practitioners, who so far lack the requisite skills. Such collaborations are now actually becoming a reality.

The History of Therapeutic Evaluation: Between Dogmatic Certainty and Empiric Probability

Ulrich Tröhler

Department of the History of Medicine,
University of Göttingen, Federal Republic of Germany

When we think of evaluating therapy today, our minds immediately turn to clinical trials. We are living in an age of clinical trials, yet because of some of their special characteristics, they are still controversial. Such trials are comparative in nature. In order to reduce observation to one parameter, others being equal, the techniques of randomization and masked assessment are used, often with the help of a placebo, and the results are described in statistical terms. These trials therefore deal with groups of patients rather than with individuals. In order to understand the present situation, it might be helpful to ask when and why these features of clinical trials were introduced, what have been the ensuing problems and what was the reaction to them at different periods of history? Finally, what was the basis for therapeutic decisions before such trials and how have decisions been influenced since?

Dogmatic or empiric?

The medical texts of Greek and Roman antiquity contain two basic approaches to therapeutics, the dogmatic and the empiric. The *dogmatic* approach required a knowledge of the cause of the disease, because therapy could then be derived rationally. If correctly deduced, the therapy was bound to work and therefore did not need to be validated. The *empiric* approach, on the other hand, saw clinical symptoms leading directly to practical therapy regardless of any theoretical considerations. An essential feature of this approach was that the outcome had to be assessed. In order to do so, the Ancients adopted the classical empirical triad of observation, comparison of the data with the literature, and

41

conclusion by analogy.[1] This seems to us to be common sense. Today, most of us follow a middle path, using a combination of dogmatic and empiric traditions.

Until fairly recently, our knowledge of the causes of disease was largely speculative, but that did not prevent an emphasis upon dogmatism by scholarly medieval practitioners and the empiric approach to treatment, being purely practical, fell into disrepute. Knowledge was based on "certainties" derived from the wisdom of the Ancients and Divine revelation and was arrived at by scholastic deductive logic. The seventeenth century, however, brought Baconian inductive logic which provided the core of a new empiricism and made experience respectable because it could be tested by experiment. At the same time, "certainty" was displaced by "probability".

In medicine this change took longer to develop than in other fields, particularly in therapeutics. For a seventeenth century learned doctor concentrating as he was on the welfare of individuals, it was difficult to think of performing experiments with group of patients. Furthermore, in therapeutics, experience could mean many things, from adherence to mere routine, to the fallacy of relating the outcome of the illness directly to the treatment given. It was an error finally realised in the eighteenth century as "pseudo-experience".[1]

Enter therapeutic experience

We owe much of our modern therapeutic experience to eighteenth century military and naval medicine. James Lind (1716–1794), for instance, is rightly famous for a planned trial of the treatment of scurvy which he conducted on board ship in 1747, and which involved six concomitantly treated groups of two patients each. His work in the second half of the century, done at Haslar Naval Hospital, was also very important. He had more than 1,000 beds at his disposal and used this opportunity for therapeutic experimentation. He set up a truly scientific programme of clinical research and suggested that a series of non-selected observations should be the basis for decisions in therapeutics. In this we see the dawn of the idea of randomization. He also campaigned against "the habit of publishing individual successful cases only"

Lind insisted that accurate notes must be kept, for memory alone could not be trusted, and that the results of treatment should be compared with the unassisted efforts of nature in comparable patients. He understood the placebo effect and presented his results statistically, often in terms of relative mortality. From such data he aimed to derive a standard plan for treating specific diseases, though he recognised that this could not be infallible in every case, for, as he put it: "Yet more enlarged experience must ever evince the fallacy of all positive assertions in the healing art".[2]

Lind was not alone in expressing such sentiments nor in putting them into practice. We find in the British literature many reports of therapeutic evaluation using observational and experimental methods ranging from the analysis of statistical returns, via "historical controls" to planned single-blind, placebo studies.[3]

Three types of opposition

Formal opposition to this empirical and probablistic approach can be found in Paris, where two formal debates took place on the issue around 1835 in the Académie Royale des Sciences and the Académie Royale de Médicine. Pierre-Charles-Alexandre Louis (1787–1872) advanced arguments in favour of statistics in clinical medicine which were similar to those of the Eighteenth Century. The counter arguments of his opponents were of three kinds. The first group, which we may call "old school", asked: "Should our old certainty be replaced by probability? Should medicine become a gambling place? By administering the same therapy indiscriminately to groups of patients, do we not deprive the single patient of his individuality? How can the variability of biological phenomena be rendered by the constancy of figures?".

The second group of arguments were more "modern". Some of them were pragmatic, for example, when it was held that two huge groups of comparable patients would never be found, or that such trials were clinically inadequate, inasmuch as they did not reflect the daily reality of the doctor who was facing an individual and not a group of patients. Some raised ethical questions and it was suggested that trials were ethically

43

disputable insofar as the organizing doctors were interested only in the outcome of the majority. To ignore the minority seemed to show a completely anti-medical attitude.[4]

The third kind of argument was "timeless". It was that the result simply could not be believed. For instance, during the cholera epidemics in Europe in the early 1830s, some hospitals applying homoeopathic treatment showed better outcomes than hospitals which had used traditional bleeding, and this could not possibly be acceptable to conventional doctors.

Discussions on clinical statistics were resumed in Paris in the middle of the nineteenth century. A sort of compromise was arrived at. Statistics with their probabilities were all right for hygiene, epidemiology or preventive medicine. But these relatively recent disciplines were seen as being quite separate from "real" medicine, which was perceived as essentially clinical. However, this discipline itself was just about to embark on claims to new dogmatic certainty by advances in patho-physiology and bacteriology; by the introduction of new diagnostic tools (such as the stethoscope, the optical "scopes", and later, the ECG and X-rays) and by the appearance of new therapeutic possibilities such as painless antiseptic surgery.

Comparative therapeutic experimentation was practically forgotten. Statistics were being used in a one-sided way. Increasing the numbers increased the impression of certainty — a technique particularly employed in the rapidly growing area of modern surgery.[5]

The recognition of the need for proper methodology in therapeutic evaluation came up again only in our own century, particularly in Anglo-Saxon countries. The first randomization was actually performed in Britain in 1923 in an agricultural field experiment. The first group randomization in a clinical trial occurred in the United States in 1931. The first individual randomization was carried out in the British Medical Research Council's streptomycin trial in 1948. This was also the first trial strictly conducted according to the double-blind technique.[6]

This chronology of events leads us to ask, first, how the quest for validation came about in the eighteenth century, secondly, how we can explain the stagnation in the nineteenth, and thirdly what caused the methodological fan to unfold again in the twentieth century?

Stagnation and resurgence

"Medical arithmetic", as these clinical trials were called in Britain in the Age of Enlightenment, was seen as a way to de-mystify medicine, as the only means of equating the standards of clinical medicine with those of other sciences and of relating it to contemporary political and economic life. A number of intellectual stimuli were present to help. Among an elite of doctors there was a preoccupation with numbers, such as mortality statistics and census records, the welfare of groups of the population, such as workers, the military, women and children, as well as with that of individuals. This preoccupation, during the nineteenth century, strongly influenced the new disciplines of hygiene and epidemiology, which then developed quite separately from clinical medicine. In the twentieth century, a sense of social obligation has played an important role in the development of our concept of the welfare state.

Social issues were also characteristic of the medical world of the eighteenth century. If a surgeon, still a sort of craftsman, wanted to move up the social ladder and overcome the social preeminence of the learned physicians, he could show, with the help of numbers, that he could outperform them. And publication of results also helped to distinguish the true medical practitioner from quacks or from colleagues who used patent medicines, a practice which was considered unethical.

A number of medical reasons can explain stagnation in the nineteenth century, besides this preoccupation with the qualitative phenomena of health and disease. Early clinical trials had often not shown any benefit from treatment when compared with the natural course of the disease. This was very difficult to accept because doctors have a desire to be helpful and a positive belief in their ability to provide that help. There was also no need for placebos when mortality levels were high. Today, the immediate threat of death is much reduced when illness or accident occurs compared to the situation even 50 years ago. The distinction between subjective and objective results has thus

45

become much more relevant. Furthermore, Government regulatory bodies nowadays require proof of objective efficacy.

But there is also a non-medical explanation for the nineteenth century stagnation and the development of evaluative methods in the twentieth century. It is to be found in the use which was made of statistics. In the nineteenth century, statistics were concerned chiefly with mass phenomena, with correlations and regressions, rather than with the determination of the significance of differences between groups. All the relevant tests of significance were developed in England only in the early twentieth century.

Avoiding pseudo-experience

When today we discuss the problem of validation of therapy in the light of historical evidence, I believe we should attempt to overcome methodological shortcomings by improved scientific skills, for the alternative would be to fall back into an age of dogmatic pseudo-experience. It may be encouraging to bear in mind the words of William Black (1749–1829), who in his Annual Oration to the Medical Society of London said in 1788:

''Physicians have been too long running astray in speculative or frivolous employments of philosophick drudgery . . . By what clue can medical wanderers find their way through the labyrinth of prognosticks and therapeuticks, except by medical arithmetic and numbers? . . . Perhaps some would here, answer, the best authors should decide the controversy. Who are they, ancient or modern? To borrow Molière's satirical expression, Hippocrates often says Yes, and Galen flatly No. The system of medical arithmetic, although it may not shew the best mode of cure that may here after be invented, it will, however, by comparison, determine the best that has yet been discovered, or [is] in use.''

References

1 Erwin H. *Ackerknecht, Therapie von den Primitiven bis zum 20 Jahrhundert* Stuttgart: Enke, 1970. Chapters IV and V.
2 Tröhler U. Towards clinical investigation on a numerical basis: James Lind at Haslar Hospital 1758–1783. *Proceedings of the Twenty-Seventh International Congress on the History of Medicine. Barcelona 1980.* Barcelona: Academia de Ciències Mediques de Catalunya i Balears. 1981; 1: 414–9.

3 Tröhler U. *Quantification in British Medicine and Surgery 1750–1830, with Special Reference to its Introduction into Therapeutics*. London: University College, 1976.
4 Murphy T D. Medical knowledge and statistical methods in early Nineteenth Century France. *Medical History* 1981; **25**: 301–19.
5 Tröhler U. *Auf dem Weg zur physiologischen Chirurgie: Der Nobelpreisträger Theodor Kocher 1841–1917*. Basel-Boston-Stuttgart: Birkhäser, 1984. Chapters 7 and 8.
6 Lilienfeld A M. Ceteris paribus: the evolution of the clinical trial. *Bulletin of the History of Medicine* 1982; **56**: 1–18.

Science and Healing

Patrick C. Pietroni
*Department of General Practice, St Mary's
Hospital Medical School, London, NW8 8EG, UK*

Basic philosophy and concepts

The current bio-medical viewpoint of health and disease is based on a Cartesian/Newtonian view of the universe and is essentially *dualistic, mechanistic* and *reductionistic*. It has served us well for over 300 years and helped bring about many discoveries for the benefit of mankind. Its major contribution to the field of medicine has been the treatment of acute medical and surgical situations affecting individual organs and tissues. However, this model has its limitations which are now becoming apparent as we struggle to find effective approaches to the management of chronic disorders as well as the common complaints that afflict mankind.

In addition, over the last 70 years or so there has been a revolution in scientific thinking that has as yet to be integrated into the bio-medical approach to health and disease. Indeed this new science is very difficult to integrate because it challenges the basic philosophical assumptions that underpin this approach. We in medicine are living through a revolution as important as the Copernican discoveries, as critical as the Darwinian challenges and as humbling as Freud's description of unconscious processes. I believe we need to make ourselves familiar with many discoveries that form the foundations of a new map of the human condition that will surely transform the practice of medicine in the next 100 years.

To give a flavour of this new world picture, let me simply quote a few of its innovators:-

Albert Einstein
We may therefore regard matter as being constituted by the regions of space in which the field is extremely intense. There is no

49

place in this new physics both for field and matter—for field is the only reality.

Niels Bohr
The great extension of our experience in recent years has brought to light the insufficiency of our simple mechanical conceptions and as a consequence has shaken the foundation on which the customary interpretation of observations was based.

Werner Heisenberg
Nothing is more important about the quantum principle than this, that it destroys the concept of the world "sitting out there". To describe what has happened one has to cross out the old word observer and put in its place the new word participator! In some strange sense the universe is a participatory universe.

Illya Prigogine
We know we can interact with nature. That is the heart of the message I give. Matter is not inert. It is alive and active. Life is always changing one way or another through its adaptation to non-equilibrium conditions. With the idea of a doomed determinist world view now gone, we can feel free to make our fate for good or ill. Classical science made us feel that we were helpless witnesses to Newton's clockwork world. Now a science allows us to feel at home in nature.

David Bohm
Ultimately the entire universe (with all its "particles" including those constituting human beings, their laboratories, observing instruments etc) has to be understood as a single undivided whole, in which analysis into separately and independently existent paths has no fundamental status.

Those who have an ear for poetry, philosophy or Eastern literature, may have noticed the similarity between some of those statements from Nobel prize-winning scientists and the writings of visionaries.

Plotinus
See all things, not in process of becoming, but in being, and see themselves in the other. Each being contains in itself the whole

50

intelligible world. Therefore All is everywhere. Each is there All and All is each. Man as he is now has ceased to be the All. But when he ceases to be an individual, he raises himself again and penetrates the whole world.

Lao Tse
Look, it cannot be seen—it is beyond form.
Listen, it cannot be heard—it is beyond sound.
Grasp, it cannot be held—it is intangible.
These three are indefinable;
Therefore they are joined in one.

William Blake
To see the world in a grain of sand
And heaven in a wild flower
Hold infinity in the palm of your hand
And eternity in an hour.

Plato
The cure of the part should not be attempted without treatment of the whole. No attempt should be made to cure the body without the soul, and if the head and body are to be healthy you must begin by curing the mind, for this is the greatest error of our day in the treatment of the human body that physicians first separate the soul from the body.

How do these ideas affect our concept of the human condition, especially as related to health and disease? Some of the conclusions that I believe can now be drawn include:

1. The human organism is a multi-dimensional being, and at one level we are bio-energetic organisms.
2. Matter and energy are interchangeable and the primary ordering factors are not biochemical, molecular or genetic but field forces and L-fields.
3. There is an inter-connectedness between all things living/ non-living, microscopic/macroscopic. The whole is greater than the sum of its parts and the part contains the whole.
4. The linear model of cause and effect is only partly applicable to disease and health.

51

5. Consciousness plays a role in the physical universe, i.e. we each possess a powerful and innate capacity for altering both our internal and external environments.
6. Health and disease lie along a continuum and represent the organism's intrinsic state of harmony with the universe.
7. One of the primary tasks of someone entrusted to heal, be he a doctor, priest or acupuncturist, is to encourage the innate capacity of the individual in distress and help restore a state of balance and harmony.

Systems of healing—Training

In delving into the field of complementary medicine I think it may be helpful to make a distinction between *methods of diagnosis, therapeutic techniques* and *comprehensive systems of healing*. The focus of this particular presentation is on the last of these categories as represented by acupuncture, chiropractic, herbal medicine, homoeopathy and osteopathy.

The legitimate and major concern for medical practitioners looking at these other disciplines is the absence of any satisfactory overall official register or criteria of competence. Here I believe the fault lies with the bodies that represent these different healing traditions. They have to provide evidence, not only that they are serious in their training schedules, but that they are willing to create a supervisory regulatory body akin to the General Medical Council. A word of caution however—professional-isation is not necessarily in the public interest. It can often become a conspiracy against the laity. It is important to provide the safeguards but not the restrictive exclusivity that comes with professionalism—for healing is everybody's business.

Let us consider the education programmes of these various schools and put them alongside medical training to see how much they have in common.

All of the training programmes maintain they focus on a whole-person approach, but looking at the curriculum I am afraid I have as much criticism of them as I have of our current medical undergraduate curriculum. There seems to be no proper interviewing course, no emphasis on illness behaviour or family dynamics, no description of the placebo response, and no attempt to focus on the health of the practitioner. Michael Balint said that the most powerful intervention (drug) a doctor can use is himself. I believe this to be true of complementary medicine as well. One of the great gaps in our current undergraduate medical curriculum is that it fails to nurture, encourage and sustain the caring, compassion and sensitivity that is essential for anyone who is entrusted to heal, no matter what his discipline. I do not know whether my colleagues in complementary medicine attempt to do this but on the published curricula I can find no direct mention of it, with the one exception of the College of Traditional Acupuncture.

Systems of healing—Research
I believe we have too much and not too little research. If we were only to implement a tenth of what we know already we would have made great progress. Secondly, in my own discipline, research and the publication of papers have for too long been accorded an importance they do not deserve. Promotion and preferment have been dictated by the length of the *curriculum vitae* over and above the human qualities of the registrar or houseman. The ability to teach, inspire and provide a role-model for students are factors that do not carry sufficient importance in academic circles.

Nevertheless, the nub of most conversations between medical practitioners and complementary therapists has been around the area of research—"prove it to me and I will believe it". The one demands the rigours of objective, clinical controlled trials with randomization and double-blind studies, whilst the other protests that the classical scientific method is not appropriate for the study of their own particular form of healing. It is difficult to enter into the debate without stereotyping and increasing the divide, but the stance that some complementary practitioners adopt—"I know because I know, because I know"— has to be challenged in the same way as the limitations of the double-blind, randomized, controlled clinical trial is now being questioned.

For me, research implies the creative pursuit of knowledge, and the scientific method as developed down the ages is only one such "method". There are other methods for attaining knowledge and the pursuit of truth—personal experience,

53

creative insights, intuitive leaps. Indeed many brilliant scientists attest to the latter methods for their most original discoveries.

Nevertheless, for the majority of us in medicine, the test as to whether a theory is scientific or not has been shaped by the observations put forward by Karl Popper. Popper's main contribution was to turn the "what is truth?" debate on its head and state that the method of science is not the gathering of evidence, but conjecture, hypothesis and refutation. He writes "the criterion of the scientific status of a theory is its falsifiability, or refutability or testability".

There has been extensive debate as to whether Popper's view of science is appropriate for the study of human beings and indeed whether we in medicine can truly be "scientific" at all. Nonetheless, it is true to say that the double-blind controlled trial is the apotheosis of British medical thinking and it certainly has been heavily influenced by the theories of Popper.

But because we live in a participatory universe; because the notion of objective knowledge is difficult to sustain, (especially as it relates to human beings); because the majority of us recognise that penicillin given with love works better than penicillin given in haste; because healing implies more than just treatment—it is difficult to justify this Chinese-box approach to the study and comparison of various forms of therapy. It is not that the truths revealed by these studies are incorrect. It is that they only provide part of the truth. We cannot use the classical methods of scientific study that separate the therapist, the therapy and the patient, that try to control the variables and that randomize the subjects, when we are looking at such a complex model. It is as if to study the behaviour of fish, we insisted on taking them out of the water. Similarly we must avoid replacing the tyranny of a method with the folly of a dogma.

The development of the scientific method brought an end to the Dark Ages and heralded the Renaissance with all its wonders. Descartes freed us from the one true religion only to lead us inadvertently to "the one true science".

We need to develop methods of inquiry that do justice to both the subjective value of human experience as well as the objective realities of the world we live in. The challenge that we face is to move from the implied opposites of the title of this presentation *science and healing* to a proper understanding of the *science of healing*.

Selected References

The Limitations of Bio-medicine

Dubos R. *Mirage of Health*. New York: Harper and Row, 1959.
Engel G. The need for a new medical model. *Science* 1977; **196**: 129–36.
Illyich I. *Limits to Medicine*. London: Boyars, 1959.
Kennedy I. *The Unmasking of Medicine*. London: Paladin, 1983.
Knowles J. *Daedalus* 1977; **106**: 1.
McKeowan T. *The Role of Medicine*. Oxford: Blackwells, 1979.
Pietroni P. Holistic medicine. New map, old territory. *British Holistic Medical Journal* 1984; **1**: 3–13.

The New Scientific Paradigm as it Affects Medicine

Bohm D. *Wholeness and the Implicate Order*. London: Routledge and Kegan Paul, 1980.
Capra F. *The Tao of Physics*. Berkeley: Shambhala, 1975.
Capra F. *The Turning Point*. London: Wildwood House, 1982.
Dossey L. *Space, Time and Medicine*. Berkeley: Shambhala, 1982.
Kuhn T. *The Structure of Scientific Revolution*. Chicago: University Press, 1970.
Meek G W. *Healers and the Healing Process*. Illinois: Quest, Wheaton, Theosophical Publishing House, 1977.
Pelletier K. *Mind as Healer, Mind as Slayer. A Holistic Approach to Preventing Stress Disorder*. London: Allen and Unwin, 1978.
Pelletier K. *Holistic Health. From Stress to Optimum Health*. New York: Delta, 1979.
Von Bertalanffy L. *General Systems Theory*. New York: Braziller, 1968.
Wilber K, ed. *The Holographic Paradigm*. Berkeley: Shambhala, 1981.

55

Role of Research in the Rapprochement between Conventional Medicine and Complementary Therapies*

Richard D. Tonkin

*Research Council for Complementary Medicine,
London W1M 9AD, UK*

In the rapprochement between conventional medicine and complementary therapies, four questions need to be addressed. Why is research into complementary therapies necessary? What exactly is the nature of the subject to be researched, and what are the particular problems involved in doing it? Finally, what long-term benefits can be expected from a successful rapprochement between conventional medicine and complementary therapies?

The need for research

If anything is certain in this uncertain world, it is that complementary therapies are here to stay—and without doubt their use will continue to expand as the months and years go by. This being so, it surely makes good sense to foster rather than fight their development and progress. However, taking part in the management of illness carries very considerable responsibilities, and therefore anyone presuming to practise in the field should recognize the need for these activities to be researched with the object of revealing any potential hazards as well as evaluating their relative benefits—in short, to provide a measure of quality control. Furthermore, research is the only means of obtaining valid evidence upon which acceptable judgements can be based for exercising proper control over the practice of any therapeutic activity—that is, for the provision of ethical constraints.

---

* Reprinted with kind permission from the *Journal of the Royal Society of Medicine* 1987; **80**: 361–3.

Taken in conjunction with existing laws in the UK, the paucity of research evidence and consequent lack of quality controls and ethical constraints in the field of complementary medicine render the public highly vulnerable to exaggerated claims of inadequately qualified persons purporting to practise a wide variety of insufficiently tested treatments. In addition, there is a very real danger of blind faith in beguilingly soft options resulting in arbitrary rejection of the well-proven benefits of orthodox scientific practice, thereby compounding the problems of long-suffering patients and resulting in more than the occasional tragedy.

An equally important factor is the appearance of an increasing number of publications purporting to provide guidance and advice on "improvement of health", and "the curing of illness". Accompanying these is a veritable flood of articles and media presentations on the same theme by people highly skilled in the art of presentation but short on the science of verification. Some of these are couched in pseudo-biochemistry to conceal the transparencies of the argument. Of course, the majority of the material is based on an element of truth — but all too often the journalistic overlay results in a dangerous distortion of the message.

In essence, therefore, the need for research in this field stems from the absence of quality controls and ethical constraints, exposing the public to the dangers of being misled by over-enthusiastic promoters of unconfirmed options.

Nature of the subject

Before going on to consider the considerable problem of researching complementary therapies, it would be wise to remind ourselves about the essential duality of sickness and of the fundamental distinction between "illness" and "disease".

"Illness" is a purely subjective state as perceived by the patient and is heavily dependent upon the inherent variability of the individual. It bears no consistent relationship to disease. "Diseases" on the other hand are specific entities and may quite often be present in the absence of any illness whatsoever.

Conversely, "health" is by no means synonymous with the absence of disease, nor even with the absence of illness. It is essentially a matter of harmonious integration of all the body systems, maintained by the bio-regulatory functions of the neuroendocrine and psychoimmunological mechanisms. This concept of health involves recognition of the body as having self-regulatory, self-defending, self-repairing, and cell-replicatory capabilities. In actuality it is therefore a continuously self-healing organism. The ''self-healing'' concept is nothing new: Hippocrates originally expressed the idea in his well known pronouncement, *vis medicatrix naturae*. The ''healing force'' of nature invoked by Hippocrates is, indeed, a natural force. It is the energy powering a series of highly complex intracellular biochemical functions and cell replicatory activities, all coordinated by a series of endogenous bioregulatory agents — enzymes, endocrines, immunoglobulins, and neuropeptides.

This being so, there is no logical reason for not accepting that these mechanisms can be mobilized or potentiated (I prefer the word catalysed) by a variety of different therapeutic activities, systems, or techniques — including both spiritual and lay healing. That said, the catalytic influence over the natural healing capability by no means excludes the probability of complementary therapies having a measure of specific action.

The really interesting thing to me is that Hippocrates anticipated the modern concept of imbalance of homoeostasis as a cause of illness in his theory of imbalance of the four humours: blood, phlegm, black bile and yellow bile. If we substitute enzymes, endocrines, immunoglobulins, and neuropeptides for his humours, the simile is virtually exact. In fact we have now come full circle, but have scientifically definable entities, as opposed to mystical designations, to work with.

However, Hippocrates was by no means a pure humouralist any more than we are pure ''homoeostasists'', for he was fully aware of the fact that diseases could arise from alterations in the structure of the body and from external influences such as climate, seasons, etc. It is no surprise that he has been universally acclaimed as the ''Father of Modern Medicine''. What is less widely recognized is that he was also the ''Father of Research''. Knowledge, he insisted, could be acquired only by observation of the processes of nature and by deduction from ascertained fact.

The various regulatory, defensive, and reparative mechanisms operate continuously and automatically. But they are profoundly influenced by the patient's attitude, being strongly potentiated by positive states of mind such as optimism, enthusiasm and the will to get better, and conversely are inhibited by the negative emotions of anxiety, apprehension and the fear of getting worse. In one way the body thrives on positive stress; on the other hand it is inhibited by distress.

"Getting better" is a mutually participatory activity between patient and therapist, and the former must not expect—let alone demand—"to be cured", nor the latter (be he orthodox or complementary) delude himself that his particular method in itself is exclusively responsible for the recovery.

Superimposed upon this is the all-important factor of patient/therapist interaction in influencing the processes of recovery. This has been encapsulated in the famous phrase "bedside manner"—all too often contemptuously dismissed as a mere placebo effect. Placebos as a whole are by no means simply a sop to the patient, as is implied by the name. A moment's thought should suffice to recognize them for what they really are—catalysts of the bio-regulatory mechanisms. In this sense they are an invariable ingredient of any therapeutic activity, and the colour of the pill—let alone the personality of the therapist—are both important factors. All of these, i.e. individual patient response, patient/therapist interaction, and the element of placebo effect, must be taken into account when carrying out research into the clinical outcome of any therapeutic procedure.

Problems of research

Unfortunately, research in this field presents considerable problems, the first of which is really so obvious that it is surprising it has not been more widely recognized before. The plain fact is that the majority of complementary practitioners lack the necessary expertise and experience, as well as the time, material facilities and finance, to mount research projects of an adequate calibre to meet the stringent standards obligatory for commanding respect in the international arena.

The deficit is primarily due to the absence in their training establishments of the intermediate echelon equivalent to the registrar grades that exist in orthodox medical schools, and whose job specification includes the implementation of research projects under the experienced guidance of their professional mentors. In fact, research of an acceptable quality (and this is mandatory) can really only be achieved with the full and active cooperation of the established profession and of sister disciplines in academic institutions.

So in a way the rapprochement has to antedate the research, and I am happy to say that the Research Council for Complementary Medicine (RCCM) has already gained the enthusiastic cooperation of nine university centres and medical schools, which now have research projects in train.

The second problem associated with researching this area is the absence of any adequate literature access facility, comparable with that available for orthodox scientific medicine, and without which any research project is seriously compromised. A start has been made on the creation of this with the active cooperation of the British Library and financial backing from the DHSS and the Hayward Trust and a grant from the Muirhead Trust for the acquisition of the necessary hardware. In the initial stages the Centre is to be based in the British School of Osteopathy.

The third problem, and this is the most demanding one of all, is the need to reconsider the whole subject of research methodology in relation to complementary therapies. Of course existing research methodologies will continue to hold an important place, but the time is now overdue for researchers to question the validity of regarding patients as rigidly standardizable objects when attempting to evaluate any activity involving their person.[1] A participatory relationship between patient and therapist is an indispensable ingredient in any treatment situation, and when research fails to follow suit it ceases to deal with reality and not infrequently runs the risk of being frankly unethical.

Peter Reason[2] rightly uses the adjective ''experiential'' to describe the more appropriate collaborative research technique, and John Heron[1] has built up a convincing volume of experience in its use. However, it still needs further exploration and refinement in therapeutic practice, as do the markers of the various bio-regulatory mechanisms involved in any recovery process. Quantifiable changes in the immune system reflect the general state of the patient and these serve as valuable indicators for monitoring the progress or otherwise of nonspecific illness, an aspect considered in a recent review under the title *The Emerging Field of Psychoneuroimmunology*.[3] There are, of course, yet other methodologies, such as computerized psychometric questionnaires, which also merit further development.

It is predominantly in the sphere of nonspecific undifferentiated illness, i.e. homoeostatic imbalance, that the greatest potential of the complementary therapeutic systems lies, and new paradigms of research are needed for adequate assessment of these. The Medical Research Council is in agreement, and I am delighted to say that it is sharing with the RCCM the funding of a Research Fellowship for the purpose of reviewing the problem *in toto*.

Benefits of achieving rapprochement

The long-term benefits that can be expected from successful integration of properly trained, accredited and registered complementary therapists with conventional scientific practitioners are far-reaching. First, it should relieve the severely restrictive and, indeed, often crippling overload with which both the general practitioner and hospital services are faced today. Secondly it should effect substantial economies in the management of the majority of patients suffering from non-life-threatening undifferentiated illness, for whom neither expensive high technology services nor costly and potentially toxic agents are necessarily appropriate. In turn this would render these same services more readily available for the minority of patients suffering from specific disease entities for which these same services and medications are unquestionably essential.

However, the full realization of these benefits can only be brought about by way of a sustained multi-disciplinary research effort, deploying all the technical facilities and creative faculties that are available in university centres and medical schools. Hence the overriding importance of surmounting the barriers of misunderstanding and of achieving an early and lasting rapprochement between conventional and complementary therapists in the interest of patients and practitioners alike.

Research could well prove to be both the bridge and the vehicle by which a truly effective rationalization of the health services could be achieved in the not too distant future. I would even go so far as to suggest that a reciprocal partnership between conventional doctors and properly trained, accredited and registered complementary therapists could go a long way towards transforming our existing National Disease Service into a National Health Service in actuality as well as name.

References

1 Heron J, Reason P. New paradigm research and holistic medicine. *British Journal of Holistic Medicine* 1984; **1**: 80–91.
2 Reason P, Rowan J, eds. *Human Inquiry: Sourcebook of New Paradigm Research*. Chichester: Wiley, 1981.
3 Solomon G. The emerging field of psychoneuroimmunology. *Advances. Journal of the Institute for the Advancement of Health* 1985; **2**: 7–19.

Directions for Research
Highlights from the Discussions

Problems of evaluation

Dr Kendall, speaking for the Council of the Section of Epidemiology and Community Medicine of the RSM, considered that the validity of claims made by therapists must be authenticated through rigorously controlled clinical trials, according to such criteria as were recommended by the GMC and the MRC. Endorsing this view, Dr Davey called for therapists to investigate their work systematically in order to gain credibility. This was already happening. For example, the Homoeopathic Research Group was now making considerable efforts to investigate the theory and practice of homoeopathy.

Dr Fraser Steele agreed that evaluation was called for, but said it could not be done in a rigorously scientific way. The needs of many patients were often quite non-specific and required non-specific treatment, often in the form of counselling. When individuals with relatively minor psychosomatic disorders went to a complementary therapist the latter might, in effect, be acting as a psychotherapist, or at least as a lay counsellor.

Professor Baum said that members of his own Department, like many others, were well aware of the importance of the spiritual side of life in health and illness. The task of the doctor was to strive to lengthen life and improve its quality. He considered it entirely mistaken to assume that the holistic idea was the sole province of those who had "hijacked" the concept of whole person care and given it a name, as if it were a new way of treating ill people. The Cancer Research Campaign was currently studying projects on psychological factors and the effects of counselling for cancer patients. They would seriously consider any other approaches, provided that they were scientifically conceived.

Professor Watson considered that scientific research into complementary therapies hinged on the question of measurement. The group had to ask itself whether such research

65

was feasible in such non-specific illnesses. He believed that it was often not possible because there were too many unquantifiable variables for exact evaluation. Dr Tonkin, however, believed that an important outcome of these Colloquia might be an assessment of the kinds of research that would be appropriate for particular techniques. One approach could be the pragmatic one suggested by Dr Horder in which participatory "research", involving both doctors and therapists, would lead to a degree of authentication.

In the experience of Dr Patel, research into many complementary therapies did not involve the exclusive use of logic and the analytical process. She endorsed Dr Horder's suggestion and felt that scientists should be encouraged to work with healers to appreciate the value of intuitive as well as logically based knowledge. Agreeing, Dr Lewith believed that any definition of science should take account of paradigms of knowledge beside those relying wholly on logic, and analysis based on logic. Cancer could be considered as an overt disease state but it was possible that bio-energetic processes which distorted homoeostatic competence could be detected long before pathological changes. It was necessary critically to examine this type of possibility.

Approaches to research

During the Fifth Colloquium a discussion group considered the question: ''Are the current research approaches in conventional medicine appropriate to complementary therapies?''.

All members agreed that, whatever methods might be appropriate, similar high standards of research were required for the evaluation of complementary techniques as for those for conventional medicine. However, it was not clear whether current models were entirely appropriate, even for orthodox medicine. Double-blind clinical trials had recognized limitations. While some complementary therapies might be amenable to currently acceptable research methods, the vitalistic philosophies upon which others were based made them difficult to investigate. In addition, complementary practitioners often lacked the scientific training and skills necessary to understand and apply research methodology. This implied a need for collaborative efforts, with the skills of the therapist being combined with those of experienced scientists.

Although medicine had evolved excellent methods for, say, drug evaluation, there was a need for greater flexibility in research design and the acceptance of new methodologies which might accommodate the multiple factors involved in any therapeutic interaction. Investigations were currently under way in China to correlate traditional energetic concepts with modern physiology and chronobiology. The study group felt that work on personality type and cardiovascular disease gave some evidence to support the traditional concept of "pre-pathology". Undifferentiated illness should provide another model by means of which it might be possible to define appropriate terms for those patterns of dysfunction which the complementary practitioner used to reach a diagnosis.

There was general agreement that conventional research methods could be successfully applied to large areas of complementary medicine but there was a need to develop new methodologies to accommodate the non-specific and holistic perspectives of many of these treatments. Moreover, it had to be recognized that it was the patient who did the healing and that patients, whenever possible, should play an active part in any investigation and research.

In welcoming these conclusions Dr Tonkin saw research as a crucial way of validating complementary therapies and of protecting the public. Research in this area was singularly difficult. It was imperative to have the collaboration of experienced scientific research workers linked to academic departments. The Research Council for Complementary Medicine had experienced formidable difficulties in establishing suitable scientific research protocols. Nevertheless, the Council had been associated with some promising research projects.

Research in particular therapies

During the Sixth Colloquium separate discussion groups considered the question of opportunities for research in manipulative therapies, homoeopathy and medical herbalism and in acupuncture.

67

Mr Dove, reporting on the manipulative therapies group, found that therapists had certainly the will to perform research. For example, the calming effects of touch ought to be investigated. There was also a need to define more precisely the syndromes for which manipulative treatment was known to be helpful, for example, the formidable problem of what was meant by "low back pain". Without more precise definition, any comparison of the efficacy of manipulation with that of analgesics would prove immensely difficult. Perhaps the most appropriate place to start was with an assessment of observer reliability. The group also advocated the use of existing case records and prospective studies in this field, while Sir James Watt drew attention to the importance of standardization of case records, and an agreed system of data collection.

The recurrent problem of jargon and the difficulty of employing a common language were seen as the greatest hindrance to comparative studies. The multivariate nature of illness most responsive to manipulative treatment would require the expertise of experienced scientists to devise appropriate protocols and to interpret the results of clinical trials. Several recent research submissions had been refused without explanation by grant awarding bodies. This suggested that the design of relevant, scientifically approved, but appropriate research protocols must have a high priority.

The group which discussed homoeopathy and medical herbalism reached a broad consensus that research should certainly be undertaken, though Dr Gormley reported that complementary therapists would be reluctant to embark upon research involving the statistical complexities of many orthodox clinical trials. A trial of homoeopathic treatment for hay fever was currently under way and appeared to demonstrate benefit beyond that accounted for by the placebo effect. A trial on the use of homoeopathic pertussin was also being planned. The group considered that the time had now come to take into account the subjective reactions of the patient which determined his sense of well-being or of illness and whether or not this was related to underlying organic states, so that more might be done for many patients in whom no organic disease could be demonstrated.

Individual case studies should also be promoted in this area. For example, in medical herbalism, a useful approach would be to assess physiological parameters in individual patients before and after prescribing a particular remedy. The efficacy of, say, garlic would be given greater credibility if it could be shown to influence physiological responses. Spiritual well-being and its influence upon illness was considered an area of great importance, which seemed to offer no specific opportunities for research, except as one facet of the multivariate analysis already considered.

Mr Hill reported that the acupuncture discussion group had, in fact, considered protocols for research in which subjective elements could be incorporated, but it was probably too early to become involved in elaborate research programmes. A more gradual approach might prove to be necessary in order to develop a sense of mutual confidence and collaboration. There was considerable doubt about the value of seeking to explain the effects of acupuncture in terms of Western science. Some aspects of the process could not be explained, let alone investigated by such methods. However, conventional physicians in the group suggested that perhaps only 20% of their own clinical work involved the use of therapy which had been proven by scientific methods.

A particular feature of acupuncture was the existence of several different schemes. If the patient did not respond to one, another scheme of diagnosis and treatment sometimes produced a positive result. Apart from demonstrating the individuality of response to treatment, this suggested that acupuncture had an influence beyond the placebo effect. However, the patient–therapist relationship was of primary importance. In acupuncture, as in other modes of complementary therapy, the practitioner aimed to place more control in the hands of the patient.

Sir James Watt said that there was a great need to identify *specific* areas for research. A general willingness to embark on research programmes was not enough. Orthodox researchers would welcome collaboration with complementary therapists but only in well-defined areas. More ought to be said, in his view, about the findings that could be generated by researching into the records of complementary therapists. So far little effort had been made in this direction.

Beyond the placebo?

Dr Lewith observed that there was not yet enough man-power to provide a base for systematic research. At his Centre for the Study of Alternative Therapies in Southampton, it had been possible to introduce medical students. This would yield an increasing number of newly-qualified people with both orthodox and complementary training and the awareness of how to apply both forms of care to their patients. Some would doubtless seek to do research. Mr Mills said that in medical herbalism there was a particular difficulty, in that many practitioners were isolated and lacked opportunities to relate to any centralised system of clinics.

Dr Taylor Reilly maintained that the crucial barrier to be cast down was the scepticism of orthodox colleagues, who firmly believed that complementary therapies depended solely on the placebo response. In Glasgow, a two and a half year trial of homoeopathy was in progress with the precise aim of testing whether homoeopathic treatment succeeded only as a placebo. Once it had been shown unequivocally that a therapy succeeded beyond this degree of efficacy, the doors of research, collaboration and finance would be opened.

Dr Nixon believed that it was important to show whether complementary practitioners were able to influence disease or facilitate healing processes in a specific way, or whether they were simply practising as psychosocial therapists.

In the view of Dr Fisher, scepticism would not be overcome by premature research with simplistic protocols. Results obtained with rheumatic patients, some of whom showed beneficial responses irrespective of the remedy used, demonstrated the complexity of the problems facing researchers using unconventional methods. Dr Kingsley considered it was essential to ensure that the statisticians who analysed such results had a real understanding of the principles underlying the various complementary therapies and a thorough knowledge of the disease process. Orthodox and complementary perspectives about the disease process differed from each other. The way in which their respective treatments were evaluated must differ accordingly.

Dr Pietroni believed that there was a danger in pressing for systematic research too soon. It could have the effect of separating orthodox and complementary therapists, rather than bringing them closer together. The most practical solution was to create opportunities for complementary therapists to work with conventional doctors. From this collaboration, ideas for feasible research would be generated. This suggestion was welcomed by hospital consultants engaged in clinical research, who offered to help complementary practitioners with an appropriate training to achieve the necessary research skills.

Looking at the records

Mr Hutchinson believed that there was ample scope to undertake retrospective studies of the records of complementary therapists to determine which conditions were treated most frequently, what percentage of patients improved and to study their age and sex distributions.

Dr Swayne said that a number of projects were currently underway in the South West of England in collaboration with the NHS. Homoeopathic studies were addressing the control of angina, night cramps in the elderly, steroid responses in children with nephrotic syndrome and obstetric analgesia. A collaborative data-base in homoeopathy was being set up and might be flexible enough to accommodate other therapies.

Professor Tröhler remarked that it was only because one physician had time to study his personal records that the therapeutic value of digitalis was discovered. If both doctors and complementary practitioners had more opportunity to examine their records in detail, a great deal of knowledge would emerge, but clinical pressures were preventing such an important research effort.

A question of funding

Professor Eiser said that there was a danger of thinking too exclusively of trials of single therapies in single centres. What was needed was a broader and more accessible data-base providing information on evaluation studies, patient referral patterns, patient choice and diagnostic decisions. The Royal Society of Medicine could give a valuable lead here.

Dr Lewith said that no one should imagine that the Government was under any obligation to provide seed money to initiate research. No rheumatologist would consider that the DHSS should fund research into back pain. The task of starting systematic research was difficult and obtaining the money was perhaps the most difficult aspect of it.

Dr Tonkin said that the Research Council for Complementary Medicine now had links with four universities, was well-advanced in providing a data-base and devoted much of its work to methodology. It could not yet provide funding for individual research projects. However, the DHSS had actually given some funds to start the data-base and the Council had established a Research Methodology Fellowship to be taken up by Dr Taylor Reilly.

His Royal Highness the Prince of Wales observed that it would always be difficult for some people to accept that certain treatments work for some individuals, but not for others, because an individual's philosophical make-up influenced attitudes about what constituted health and illness. He was greatly encouraged by the evidence of good-will that could lead, as at Charing Cross Hospital, to more collaboration in research and practice. It was excellent that some headway was being made for the greater benefit of patients and that was obviously the ultimate objective.

Quality Control in Training and Practice

There is a major need to ensure that the training of complementary practitioners, together with the procedures and medicines that they use, are all of the highest agreed standards. Quality control of medicines is a Government responsibility. However, the certification of training and practice is more a matter for individual disciplines. It appears desirable that this should come under the aegis of some central body, with an overall monitoring responsibility, to ensure the achievement and maintenance of agreed standards of excellence.

Baroness Trumpington expresses the current Government attitude both to the registration of complementary medicines and complementary therapists. There is, she suggests, a major difference between herbal and homoeopathic remedies in terms of legislation, and homoeopathic remedies will require different methods of evaluation. It is for alternative therapists themselves to address the question of standards and qualifications.

Sir David Innes Williams considers that the medical profession can and does adapt to challenges by its competitors. A pattern of effective professional collaboration has already been provided by the relationship established between the medical profession and professions supplementary to medicine. Ultimately, it is for the complementary practitioners themselves to set standards of education and competence which will win the confidence both of the medical profession and the public, and that will largely determine any future relationship with the National Health Service.

Alternative Medicines and Therapies and the DHSS*

Baroness Trumpington
*Parliamentary Under Secretary of State, Department
of Health and Social Security, London SE1 6BY, UK*

The last few years have seen an increasing awareness that the whole patient needs to be treated as much as the diseased organ or system of the body. It seems to me that the holistic approach is one that can and should be employed by all forms of medicine. Terms frequently used to describe forms of health care outside the mainstream of "conventional" medicine include "holistic", "complementary" and "alternative". I prefer the term "alternative", not for dogmatic reasons, but because I feel a little uneasy about the idea of herbal or homoeopathic medicines "complementing", say, an antibiotic. One has to recognize that within the so-called umbrella term of alternative therapies is a wide range of possible treatments. Many procedures are only regarded as "alternative" when the claims for their use are greatly extended; for example manipulative therapy for a severely deformed rheumatoid joint. Other therapies derive from differing philosophies and have to be seen in their historical context.

Individual freedom

As might be expected, my approach to the subject of alternative medicine is political rather than medical and derives largely from my views about individual freedom, because I believe that our collective attitude to individual freedom is important in this context.

The traditional view of individual freedom is that we can do what we like provided we do not interfere with the freedom of others. To enable such an objective to be achieved, by common

* Reprinted with kind permission from the *Journal of the Royal Society of Medicine* 1987, **80**: 336–8.

consent we have to agree to some rules for individual behaviour. Thus the freedom of the individual is curtailed to optimize the freedom of all. For example, I accept the restriction that requires me in the UK to drive on the left-hand side of the road in the knowledge that the absence of such a rule would seriously interfere with my freedom and everyone else's to travel safely on the highway. This ingrained habit may, of course, have a reverse effect on those who cross my path when (and in this context only, I speak for myself) I cross the Channel into Common Market countries.

All this is a considerable over-simplification, but it illustrates the framework within which the Government seeks to intervene from time to time to maintain our freedoms. Some say it is legislation that holds the framework together. I like to think there is more to social cohesion than law but, that aside, one of the favourite issues for debate is the question of how much law do we need? You hear it everywhere: "There should be a law against it." At the same time the imposition of authority is often greeted with the remark, "It's a diabolical liberty." So we want freedom of action and freedom of choice and we want to be protected but not over-protected.

Translated into health care terms, these requirements manifest themselves in a breathtaking variety of legal requirements, professional standards and ethics and idiosyncratic customs. To a very large extent, the liberation view—"It's my body and I'll do what I like with it"—is upheld. Certain perverse habits are forbidden, but generally we can abuse our bodies while we are in good health, ignore good advice when we are ill and refuse treatment if we do not want it. What the law and professional bodies *are* concerned with, however, are the quality and effectiveness of the people and products involved in health care. If we are ill and we seek treatment—and most people do—then we want to be protected from unsafe and ineffective medicines, and beyond that we wish to be protected from the charlatan and from fraudulent claims. I would suggest that it is only if we can be protected from such excesses that it is possible for us to retain a genuine freedom of choice.

On the face of it that conclusion seems unobjectionable, but it does conceal three important assumptions—namely, that all illnesses can be accurately diagnosed, that all conditions can be

76

treated and that all treatments are effective. I am sure no one would accept those three assumptions as valid. Indeed, against a background of high public expectation, all health care practitioners are aware of the difficulty of conveying the message to a seriously or chronically sick person or his nearest and dearest that—to put it at its simplest—they do not have all the answers and indeed may have nothing further to offer the patient. For many unwell people it is a question of aspiration—the desire for recovery—and achievement—the body's ability to respond, and of how the gap between the two is filled. I would like to return to this concept later because I believe it offers some clues as to the reasons why alternative medicines and therapies exist, and indeed why they are necessary.

From what I have said, it will come as no surprise to anyone to know that I wholeheartedly support the freedom of the individual to seek the benefits of alternative medicines and therapies. This is a view I share with other Health Ministers and it has been repeated on a number of occasions. It is very easy to speak in support of a cause that has a strong popular following. But Health Ministers have certain formal responsibilities about medicines which call for much more than simply voicing our support. I shall therefore describe those responsibilities as they apply to alternative medicines and also say something about what might be called our informal responsibilities as regards alternative therapies, and will close with a personal view of why I think alternative care is necessary.

The Medicines Act and alternative medicines

The distinction between medicines and therapies is important because all medicines, including alternatives, come under the Medicines Act, whereas there is no equivalent legislation for the therapies. To state the obvious, the main alternative medicines are herbals and homoeopathics. They are different from each other in two important respects: homoeopathics are usually presented in highly diluted form, but herbals are not; and secondly, homoeopathics are usually sold without indications, whereas herbals are invariably labelled as suitable for treating specific conditions. These differences are significant when considering how the requirements of the Medicines Act are applied.

77

All medicines—conventional and alternative—that were on the market when the Medicines Act came into force in 1971 were given licences of right. Nothing was done at that time to check them for safety, quality and efficacy—the basic requirements for a Medicines Act licence. The intention was that over the following years this would be done by the DHSS as the Medicines Act Licensing Authority. Good progress has been made. Of the 39,000 medicines on the market in 1971, about 15,000 remain to be reviewed. Many of the original 39,000 were withdrawn, usually voluntarily by the manufacturer because they had outlived their usefulness.

Effort in reviewing these old medicines has concentrated on the more powerful conventional medicines and only in the past year have we started to look at alternatives. Early action has of course been taken when safety issues have arisen and questionable alternatives have been examined and, where appropriate (Sassafras, for example), removed from the market.

Herbal remedies

Over the next few years we expect to review some 700 herbal products. The DHSS approach is pragmatic. Many herbals are sold without prescription for minor self-limiting conditions such as coughs, colds, rheumatic pains, indigestion, headaches, etc. In the case of products for these sorts of condition we shall not press for evidence from clinical trials and pharmacological tests. Full account will be taken of the traditional nature of these products and manufacturers will be expected to support applications for reviewed licences with references from the literature of their remedial use. While we are looking for no more than an appropriate level of proof of efficacy, manufacturers will need to satisfy the DHSS as licensing authority that the products are absolutely safe and that the quality of manufacture is completely satisfactory. In applying these arrangements, herbal products are treated no differently from conventional, well-established, over-the-counter products.

Herbal products for more serious conditions such as high blood pressure and depression call for a different approach. These are conditions where the intervention of a doctor is necessary and, in fairness to both doctor and patient, it is right that full proof

78

of efficacy should be demonstrated before a licence is granted. At first, manufacturers of herbal products were worried by what they saw as unnecessarily stringent requirements. Officials at the DHSS have worked closely with the representatives of these manufacturers, and the rationale of our approach is now understood and accepted. Where therapeutic claims cannot be substantiated, officials will discuss with manufacturers the modification of these claims to a level commensurate with the evidence available. By this means I expect most herbal products to remain on the market but with unsubstantiated claims removed. As a result, on completion of the review, consumers will be able to choose from the herbal remedies on sale with increased confidence about their safety and their effectiveness for the conditions given on the packet label. In this way the review will *increase* the freedom of the consumer to exercise an informed choice.

Homoeopathic remedies
As mentioned earlier, these are significantly different from herbals. I would venture to say that herbals have more in common with modern pharmaceuticals than with homoeopathics, although the two are classed as alternative medicines. Such is the nature of classical homoeopathic care, with its highly diluted remedies and prescriptions related not to the condition but to an analysis of the whole patient, that I foresee problems when applying the Medicines Act to these remedies. The Act is built around the concept that a particular medicine has a particular purpose or set of purposes. Consequently a medicine's effectiveness can be judged against the extent to which that purpose is achieved. In accordance with homoeopathic philosophy, a practitioner might treat the same condition in two patients with entirely different medicines. He might treat two different conditions in two patients with the same medicine. His decision in each case would depend on his analysis of the whole patient. I am not qualified to debate the validity of this approach but it does present a difficulty when the Medicines Act licenses of right for homoeopathic remedies come to be reviewed—which would certainly not be for several years—or when new licences for homoeopathics are applied for.

One possible solution is that, before the review is set in motion, we introduce a modified form of licensing for homoeopathics which deals only with the safety and quality of the ingredients and the acceptability of the method of manufacture. The question of efficacy would be left to the professionals and the patient would look to the prescribing doctor or to the pharmacist for advice. The fact that homoeopathic products do not fit easily into the Medicines Act pattern has to be faced and I am sure a satisfactory arrangement can be evolved. Over the next year or so the DHSS will consult widely on the matter and the views of professional bodies, manufacturers and associations and others will be very welcome.

Freedom of choice and consumer protection

One of the themes I have tried to develop is the relationship between freedom of choice and consumer protection. The trick is to get the balance right; just enough of the one so as not to reduce the other to an unacceptable level. The licensing arrangements under the Medicines Act illustrate how we try to ensure that a wide choice of medicines is available which are safe and effective. Yet no such arrangement exists in respect of alternative therapies. Some people argue that it is the Government's responsibility to register alternative therapists. It may come to that one day, but if it does it will be because the alternative community has been unable to put its own house in order.

In principle I am against Government interference in this area. There is an essential difference between medicines which are regulated, and therapies which are not. Medicines are consumed and once consumed the arrangements for reversing the process if the product is unsafe can be very distressing for the patient; so the medicine must be safe—hence the licensing requirement. In the case of most therapies the patient can withdraw and seek other advice if he is not satisfied. Usually no harm is done, but I recognize this may not always be the case—especially if effective treatment is seriously delayed as a consequence.

I am firmly of the view that alternative therapists must themselves address the question of standards and qualifications. Many arguments have been put forward for limiting freedom to practise — perhaps through the use of registers. One argument is the danger that alternative therapy could attract charlatans and get-rich-quick merchants. But the alternative community is sensitive to this possibility, and I do not think it is yet a compelling argument to limit freedom to practise. Another reason for registration is professional status — a worthy aim, but one that alternative practitioners must convince society they deserve. A problem that prevents the further development and acceptability of alternative therapies is the super-abundance of organizations concerned. To the outsider they all seem to be making similar claims and have common objectives. This can only confuse the public. I have myself been active in encouraging representative bodies to meet each other to see what scope there is for them to ''get their act together'' — a phrase that was used many times in the debate on alternative therapies in the House of Lords in 1985. If the organizations representing alternative practitioners are going to get their message across then they need unison or harmony, but not discord.

There is no doubt that some people want alternative medicines and therapies and while this is the case they will continue to flourish. No Government is going to ban them, although I believe it is right that the medicines should be controlled to ensure, first, that they are not harmful and, secondly, that sick people are not led astray by unsupported claims of cures for — in particular — serious illnesses. Patients with diabetes, for example, or parents concerned about preventing whooping cough, should not be lured away from well established and proven and conventional methods of treatment. As to therapies, we also have to ensure that the therapists' representative bodies should set and maintain high standards of practice. I am hopeful that this will happen without Government intervention.

The case for alternative medicine

While I think that most doctors are content to live with the existence of alternative medicines and therapies, and indeed some find them a useful aid in patient care, there are doctors who are unhappy at the lack of scientific proof of efficacy. This view is exemplified in the recent report of the British Medical Association's Board of Science and Education. It would be reasonable for such doctors to ask why all this energy, both public and private, is being expended on these so-called therapies and medicines when there is little or no evidence that they work? I shall try to answer that question by reference to the point I made earlier about the gap between what is needed to achieve recovery and what in fact can be done by the doctor, and by reference to the BMA's report itself.

The BMA's report helps us to identify the sort of people who turn to alternative care. They are those who are suffering from self-limiting minor conditions who are a little frightened of modern medicines. Provided they took reasonable care of themselves, these patients would get better in time. The alternative medicine provides some comfort on the way and may not actually contribute to recovery. I can see great difficulty in mounting clinical trials to prove the efficacy of the medicine in such circumstances. Then there is the patient with the undiagnosable condition for whom conventional medicine does not seem to be able to help. So the patient turns to alternative therapy or medicine. The third category is the patient whose condition is diagnosed but who is not responding to treatment. In this category we can also include the patient for whose condition there is no satisfactory treatment; the condition is not necessarily terminal, just untreatable.

What are the people in my second and third categories to do? Many, most perhaps, persevere with orthodox care and get some relief although they are not cured. For some this is not enough and they turn to alternative therapies. The fact that these therapies are not scientifically proven is not a consideration when such decisions are made. What these patients are looking for is hope. This is what fills the gap when modern medicine is unable to achieve what the patient wants. This is not the only solution. Some are sustained by religious belief, some by a personal toughness of spirit.

The fact that the gap does exist is no criticism of modern medicine. The gap is narrowing. The BMA's report is right to remind us of the great achievements of medical science in the Twentieth Century and at the same time to warn us against expecting too much of modern technological development.

One statement in the report made me ponder on what it is that makes people tick when they are ill, with no apparent hope of full recovery:

"It is sometimes argued that it is cruel to try to dissuade a patient suffering from a condition for which there is no known cure, such as some degenerative conditions of the nervous system, from undergoing some unusual and often expensive course of treatment, on the grounds that it deprives him of hope. Against this it may be the duty of the doctor to point out that the money involved might be better employed, for example, in modifications in the house to lessen the effects of disability."

This is a humane, rational and sensible piece of advice and is the right course of action for some people. It may also be seen as the holistic approach to the patient and his illness. But it is not right for everyone. Alternative medicines and therapies may or may not deliver relief or satisfaction but they provide hope for some people. I think that is very important.

In a thoughtful letter published recently in *The Times*, one correspondent, referring to orthodox and alternative treatment, said: "What a pity we cannot just calmly and carefully assess everything and keep the best of both worlds". That may be a tall order, but it is a commendable objective and I believe that the Royal Society of Medicine's initiative in arranging their Colloquia on Conventional Medicine and Complementary Therapies is an important step in discovering the best of the alternative world.

Non-medical Professionals:
Complementary or Supplementary?

Sir David Innes Williams
Imperial Cancer Research Fund, Lincoln's Inn Fields,
London WC2A 3PX, UK

It is agreeable on occasions such as the Colloquia to be anodyne; to see this superficial disputation as having a fundamental unity of purpose; to look to the time when all purveyors of medical care will perceive the value of the others, agree on a basic pathology and achieve a genuine complementarity; when all the groups represented here will have a recognized programme and a system of registration by which the public can recognize the fully qualified practitioners of those arts. And much of the sweet reasonableness that has been displayed would encourage that view.

Problems with cooperation

I think, however, that things may not be quite so easy, and that cooperation will not be readily forthcoming. We learn from Holland that cooperation there has rested not on scientific proof but on political and social willingness. This is made clear in the chapter by Dr van Es (p. 99). And I think we have to recognize this fact. Health care in its broadest sense is a popular commodity for which there is a ready market. Those who seek to meet this demand are basically in competition with one another, and to talk of ''complementary'' rather than ''alternative'' medicine is in some areas dangerous and conceals a basic rivalry.

Of course, we can live with a certain amount of competition. It's healthy, they say—and occasionally convenient. But there are limits. And I think that is also true of conventional medicine. The established medical profession can and very well may adapt, in spite of the incredulity with which that statement will be greeted in certain quarters.

85

I am actually very impressed by the way the medical profession has altered over the course of years and has taken quite different concepts into its basic philosophy. I do like the idea that a manipulative treatment should very well be included in the skills to be acquired by some medical practitioners. I see no reason against it. In fact, Paget, that great surgeon of the Nineteenth Century actually invited the medical students at St Bartholomew's Hospital to listen to the bone-setters and even acquire some of the skills of the plasterers, though unfortunately most orthopaedic surgeons did not take his advice. I see no reason why Dr Nixon's students should not appreciate the need to teach their patients about preventing further coronary problems as well as referring them to a surgeon for by-pass surgery as he makes clear in the discussion on International Collaboration (p. 122). It does not seem to me that it necessarily needs a separate profession in order to introduce that skill.

It does the medical profession good to be told about these things, and the medical profession does change. In fact, most of the medicine and surgery in London was itself a reaction against the establishment. The specialist hospitals of this City were actually set up by competitors who could not stand the orthodox regime of the Middlesex, St Peter's Hospital and the like. They were the rebels of that time.

Philosophy and practice
We ought to look at the ways in which there could be a unifying trend. Can we understand one another's philosophy? I do not believe in "black magic". I think that if a method of treatment is effective, we ought to be able to find out why it is effective. If acupuncture works—and there seems to be good evidence that it does—then I would want to know in terms of basic biology or of basic psychology why it works, and what else I can do with that information. I think that we ought to be able to work towards a common pathology, but I do not see very much sign of it at the moment.

Can we work together in practice? Obviously, at times, we can. But I think we have to recognize that there will be a good deal of opposition. Some of the present professions supplementary to medicine are those with which, on the whole, doctors work

86

well (some of them are independent professions like chiropodists who may well deal with patients entirely in their own capacity). Some of them are also professions which have patients referred to them by the doctors. The physiotherapist in a hospital is in that category. But I am not sure whether chiropractors and osteopaths would be prepared simply to take patients who had been referred to them from doctors. Medico-legal problems may arise with regard to questions of collaboration and supervision, but they already do in regard to nurses and physiotherapists. I think it is not totally impossible to find a solution to that difficulty.

The same cooperation, of course, can occur in general practice. But if we have this sort of cooperation, there must certainly be an accepted professional standard of education and some certification of competence. There has been some discussion about an ''alternative General Medical Council (GMC)'', and whether the present Council for Complementary and Alternative Medicine is an embryo body that could act in this way. But one has to remember that the GMC was actually aiming to bring together a number of educational bodies whose qualifications sought to produce the same profession—clinical doctors. They were not intending to produce acupuncturists or osteopaths. I think that this makes a great difference.

The lesson of history?

We might also look at what happened to dentists. The licence in dental surgery, the first professional qualification, was set up in 1858 at the same time as the GMC, indeed by the same Act. To begin with it made very little difference. There were relatively few licentiates and it was not until the 1870s that the term ''dentist'' or ''dental surgeon'' was restricted to those who had a qualification. But even that did not produce a great change because people called themselves something else. In spite of the fact there were many University courses in dentistry, and a lot more qualified dentists, there were still a great number of amateurs. A lot of teeth were pulled and a lot of sockets were filled. The situation continued to be unsatisfactory until the 1920s when the Dentists. Act made it illegal for anyone other than a qualified dentist or doctor to practise dentistry.

This is a salutary story but I cannot see medicine going that way. I cannot see that we should ever have a Legislative Act which would make it illegal to practise medicine unless you are either a qualified doctor or, for example, a qualified osteopath, because a certain freedom of choice is something we regard as our birthright in this Country. But unless you have a sufficient number of practitioners who are trained to satisfy the demand totally, you will still have what in the construction industry are called the "cowboys". I think that this is a great danger for the practitioners of alternative medicine. Although some of them may receive a very satisfactory education and have a very ethical practice, there are still going to be, in the public mind, similarities between them and someone who merely puts up his plate and advertises in the local press.

Competition by price?

Of course, in the United States, the osteopaths are already recognized. I suspect that this is a reflection of the fact that the USA has a very large market and the conventional physicians have placed so high a price on their product that there is ample scope for some competitors. Whether this could happen in the UK where, with the NHS, the problem is not price but scarcity, is not clear. But I do easily foresee a time when, if trained osteopaths were so numerous and had demonstrated their skills so often to the public, there might be a public demand for inclusion of their services under the National Health Service. Whether osteopaths would be better off in that circumstance I am not at all sure, and I do think that there is a great deal to be done before that point is reached.

I do not believe it sufficient simply to discuss the problem with the Department of Health. In order to move forward it is also necessary to convince the rest of the medical profession, because the medical profession is still a powerful lobby with the DHSS and still represents votes. This, as Sir James Watt has said, is not just a question of scientific proof. It is a question of politics as well and that, I am afraid, is the reality that we have to face.

Quality Control in Training and Practice
Highlights from the Discussions

Lowering of standards
Dr Whittet said that a law enacted by Henry VIII still applied, enabling anyone to seek treatment from anyone who claims to be able to provide it. The pharmacist (formerly the apothecary) was very often the first contact made by the patient with "the greater medical profession". More work could be done by pharmacists, provided that there were proper precautions to avoid mis-diagnosis or delay.

Sir James Watt noted that the Medical Act of 1511 was a true reforming measure designed to eliminate unqualified practitioners of fringe medicine. The pressure of public opinion however caused the King to amend this Act in 1543 to enable anyone to practise. This led to an immediate lowering of standards.

Medical student education and complementary therapies
During the Fifth Colloquium a group considered the question "Should we make medical students more aware of the potential of complementary therapies, and if so, how?"

Reporting for the discussion group, Mr Lambert said that they had agreed that all medical students should be given information by complementary therapists themselves about their philosophy, scope and methods, but that no students should be taught the techniques of complementary therapy since undergraduates had enough information to assimilate in their own studies. Only those complementary therapies with a recognized training period and qualification by which the practitioner was registered with a professional body should be involved in such a programme. The first exposure should occur as early as possible and before the student was too far into his clinical studies. The potential of complementary therapies should be explored within the clinical experience of the medical students. Discussion of the appropriateness of complementary therapies might occur during

89

ward rounds and students might see such practices being applied, as in Dr Nixon's Department at Charing Cross Hospital.

It was also felt that trainee GPs should be given information about complementary therapies and be encouraged to gain first-hand experience of such procedures. This already happened through the General Council and Register of Osteopaths and individual members of that Register.

None of the group dissented from the view that complementary therapy should be incorporated into medical undergraduate experience and the general consensus was that medical students would become better practitioners as a result.

Dr Peters, speaking as a GP trainer, felt that the pre-training GP period was not ideal. This was a time when young doctors were already considerably stretched in making the transition from hospital to the general practice environment, but Dr Lewith said that, in his experience, it was possible to do a great deal in two or three morning seminars. The amount of time required was not a major constraint.

Professor McColl thought that a great mistake in contemporary medical training was early specialisation. He suggested that the principles of complementary therapy should be introduced in teaching from the outset and thereafter throughout the student's training.

It was generally agreed that a GP should only practise a particular complementary therapy after he had embarked on the long training involved, but knowledge of the principles of complementary therapies was another matter entirely. Such principles should be clearly grasped so that the significance of different approaches and their potential applications could be properly appreciated.

Freedom of choice and consumer protection

During the Seventh Colloquium a discussion group considered the question "How can freedom of choice and consumer protection be reconciled?". Mr Breen, summarizing the discussion, said that the group had been surprised to learn that manipulative therapies had seemed to be less concerned about standards of practice than others, such as herbalism or homoeopathy. Too much legislation in other countries should not act as a deterrent to necessary legislation in the United Kingdom. The question had been asked, "What are we protecting people from?" and the answer must be that the public required protection from serious accidents, including fatalities. A parallel was drawn with anaesthetics, in which the non-registration of anaesthetists was unthinkable.

Some discussants felt that State Registration might be needed, particularly in the area of manipulation. However, it was argued that doctors utilising complementary techniques were subject to no effective quality control in the practice of the complementary therapies they employed, despite General Medical Council (GMC) surveillance. In the matter of freedom of choice, GPs might be seen as health brokers with a wide knowledge of the options available to those seeking help from complementary practitioners, but there were doubts about a GP's impartiality. This could compromise the public's freedom to choose the therapy which might suit the patient best. It was also suggested that it might be a help to keep the DHSS aware of the changing policies of representative bodies of the various therapy organizations.

In summary, the group believed that the principle of a patient's freedom of choice should be upheld; that therapy organizations should maintain comparable standards and that mutual respect and cooperation should exist across the heterodox/orthodox divide, with access to records a matter for urgent consideration. The Council for Complementary and Alternative Medicine was itself embarking on a self-validation programme and others might wish to follow.

Need for an umbrella organization?
A second group considered the question "How should common educational standards and clinical practice be achieved through an umbrella organization?". Its spokesman, Dr Taylor Reilly reported that it was not clear that such an organization should exist, nor that it had a useful role. The Council for Complementary and Alternative Medicine (CCAM), which in February 1985 brought together eight main organizations, might be the model for such a body.

If the umbrella organization had an educational function, it could then help individual therapies to achieve the academic

91

goals that they had set for themselves. It might initiate a four-year course in basic healing skills, although such a time period might prove to be inadequate. However, such an umbrella body should be primarily concerned with ethics and safe practice before tackling common educational standards. It seemed clear, from Baroness Trumpington's remarks, that the therapies could expect little external help in "getting their act together" as she had put it. Concern was also expressed that an umbrella organization might merely invite orthodoxy to move in and take over. However, the complementary therapies had already seen how the attitude of the Medical Research Council had changed. It now saw medicine in its broadest sense and was prepared to channel funding towards new and hitherto unexplored areas. Perhaps in time the GMC would do the same.

The discussion ended on a note of caution. Some complementary practitioners feared that a GMC of "orthodox–alternative professionals" might try to close the door on the common law right in Britain to practise healing and caring which had allowed complementary medicine to reach its present stage of development.

Complementary medicine and the NHS

A third group considered the question "Has complementary and alternative medicine a viable role within the NHS?". Dr Lewith reported that it was considered feasible to have complementary practitioners in the National Health Service. However, they foresaw problems. The first was the legal situation. Could such practitioners make decisions about the clinical management of patients? The second was money. The DHSS was clearly not going to provide funds for any such attachment. Baroness Trumpington said that funding was now in the hands of consultants, hospital units and the Family Practice Committees and that the financial implications of clinical decisions were being handed back to the doctors.

Nevertheless, in the area of primary care, it was suggested that complementary practitioners might be brought in under the 70% reimbursement schemes now being used to bring counsellors into general practice. Under such circumstances, what would their function be? Would the osteopath be seen as "someone else who deals with bad backs", or would he have a much broader role? Would the acupuncturist deal only with pain? The answers would largely depend upon the outcome of relevant medical education, both at undergraduate and postgraduate level.

In two instances where complementary therapists were involved in hospital work, at Hackney and at Charing Cross, they had freedom to make their specific contributions to the team. There were other models in different parts of the country and we had much to learn from them all. In collaboration of this sort Mr Goodman recognized that a fundamental difference of basic philosophy between the orthodox and complementary practitioners made it difficult for doctors to accept alternative therapies easily. For instance, orthodox emphasis in preventive medicine might be on immunization and sanitation, while complementary practitioners were concerned with other aspects of the environment that caused illness such as diet, personal relationships and the home and work environment.

Consumerism and the law

Dr Kendall wondered whether complementary therapists in law took on full responsibility for the patients' treatment. In reply, Mr van Straten stated that there was no doubt that all alternative and complementary therapists were liable in law for their actions. Reputable bodies within complementary medicine were covered by their own private insurance schemes. The less reputable could not get insurance cover. He agreed that the DHSS would not consider funding until the complementary therapies established a central organization that would speak with authority on questions of standards.

Mr Laitey wondered about the legal position of complementary therapists working with an orthodox physician. He asked whether a mistake made by an osteopath would place legal responsibility on the physician with whom he was working. Mr Sandler said that if a GP referred a patient to him, that patient was informed that Mr Sandler was now responsible for his case. If he returned the patient back to the doctor, the doctor re-assumed responsibility and it was important to make the position entirely clear to the patient. Mr van Straten emphasized

93

that all alternative and complementary therapists were liable in law for their actions and all reputable bodies were covered by private insurance schemes.

Dr English saw that homoeopathy would be at a special disadvantage by the application of the Medicines Act. It would be impossibly difficult to produce evidence of efficacy using orthodox scientific methods. Sir James Watt's understanding of Lady Trumpington's remarks was that homoeopathy would indeed need special consideration. But she had made no positive assertion about the way in which the Medicines Act would be applied to the assessment of homoeopathic remedies.

Dr Kendall believed that the DHSS would want evidence of efficacy of all complementary therapies. Such evidence was largely lacking at present, but when it became available there was no reason to suppose that the DHSS would not accept it. Mr Mills however considered that the DHSS was far more concerned to protect the public than to seek proof of the efficacy of treatment. He felt Lady Trumpington had implied that if complementary practitioners did not ''get their act together'', they could expect to be subjected to regulation. However, it was extremely difficult for therapists to organize themselves effectively if there were no statutory authority to provide a framework for that coordination.

Areas of uncertainty

Dr Lewith felt that it was vital to discover what the British people wanted with respect to complementary medicine. The CCAM might find it fruitful to work with the Consumers Association which was mounting an epidemiological study. There were millions of consultations with complementary therapists but the actual data were flimsy. Dr McDonald agreed. There was strong pressure to incorporate osteopathy within the NHS, but the delay was being caused by a lack of scientific evidence. Unfortunately the DHSS would not commit resources to provide such evidence.

As Chairman of the CCAM, Mr Mills said that, within the next five years, there might be a doubling or trebling of public demand for complementary therapies. However, the CCAM had no pretention to represent itself as an umbrella organization.

94

He saw it more as a "collective" in which he hoped that the full integrity of the constituent bodies would be maintained.

Mr Sandler reiterated that there were about 900 osteopaths on the Register. The total would be about 5000 if others not on the Register were included. He believed that collaboration, initially at least, would have to be at the local level. The training of registered osteopaths would have to be considerably increased to meet the increasing national demand for competent therapists in this field.

Dr Gilbertson believed that once the public became aware that complementary therapists were well trained and capable there would be an ever mounting demand for their services to be made available within the NHS. However, Dr Lewith suggested that it should not be assumed tacitly or explicitly that all complementary practitioners necessarily wanted to become associated with conventional colleagues.

International Collaboration

In studying the question of how complementary practitioners might come to be better accepted, and how greater collaboration with orthodox medicine can be achieved in the United Kingdom, we have much to learn from experience in other countries. Recent events in the Netherlands, South Africa and the United States are all discussed. Similarly, a knowledge of such practices abroad may provide the foundation for practical programmes of collaboration at an international level.

J. C. van Es describes how over 5000 practitioners offer some form of alternative therapy in the Netherlands. In general their relationship with orthodox practitioners is good. Indeed, many of them are themselves general practitioners, but the therapies he describes cover a much broader spectrum than the limited number of complementary therapies represented in the Colloquia.

However, the distinction between the orthodox and the complementary is much more rigid in South Africa, as H. C. Gaier explains. By skilful organization a number of complementary therapies formed themselves into the Associated Health Service Professions, a legally recognized governing body which itself sets exacting standards for the six-year, full-time academic training course which recognized practitioners must follow.

In the United States, the majority of consultations are now covered by health insurance. Robert Duggan discusses this rise in the popularity of complementary therapies against the background of preventive health care as it has emerged in the USA in the last decade.

Conventional Medicine and Complementary Therapies in the Netherlands

J. C. van Es

Department of General Practice, Free University of Amsterdam, Netherlands

In the history of medical practice in the Netherlands the year 1865 is one of the most important milestones. After 20 years of preparation, four bills were passed into law. In one of these four laws the qualifications of medical doctors were regulated; a second law regulated medical practice. The result was that the right to practice medicine was exclusively conferred upon those who, after following a revised medical curriculum in university and university hospital, had passed a medical State Examination to practice medicine, surgery and obstetrics. By the introduction of this new qualification the problem of the great diversity among medical practitioners seemed to be solved. From that moment on, the 32 different types of licensed medical practitioners no longer existed.

In 1848, seventeen years earlier, the Dutch Medical Association had been founded. It is understandable that this professional organization was strongly in favour of the new law. Medical doctors received a monopoly to examine and treat patients. From that time, treatment by others was illegal and could be condemned. In the meantime the concept of the complete doctor, qualified to do everything in medical practice, was undermined by the start of specialization in medicine. The full qualification still existed in law, but was modified by regulations of the Dutch Medical Association, under which tasks and responsibilities were divided between specialists in different disciplines. Exceeding the barriers of what is customary in this division of work was to be condemned in medical courts.

Fringe areas of medicine

In spite of this traditional division, the Dutch Medical Association in 1975 devoted its Annual Scientific Congress to what

99

was called the *fringe areas of medicine*. It was the first time the official medical organization had discussed this very touchy subject in public. In an introductory statement the choice of this theme was explained: ''. . . the fact that therapies like acupuncture, homoeopathy and anthroposophic medicine exist and are a social reality, because patients seek help in alternative medicine [the name for these and other forms of non-academic medicine in the Netherlands], made it unrealistic to neglect them, notwithstanding the fact that many doctors had—and still have—very negative feelings about alternative medicine.''

Why this choice of topic? In the mid 1970s many medical students became very interested in alternative forms of medical treatment and I am sure that this Congress of the Dutch Medical Association was one of the reasons why a Government Committee was formed to study the significance and consequences of alternative therapies in the Netherlands. As a result of the report which it produced, the State Secretary of Health asked the National Health Council to advise him on the legal, financial and other consequences of alternative therapies. A new law on medical practice is also in preparation, according to which it will no longer be the exclusive right of medical doctors to treat patients.

I will try to provide a picture of the situation today in relation to alternative therapies although it is impossible fully to give reliable figures, because there is no official registration of alternative therapies. The existing data are collected by order of the State Commission on Alternative Therapies, by the Health Council and by personally interested doctors and sociologists. Sources for these statistics are membership rolls of organizations in alternative therapies and interviews with key persons, so their precision is in considerable doubt.

The Netherlands have rather more than 14.5 million inhabitants. There are over 9400 practising specialists and over 5600 general practitioners. There are more than 3000 ''organized'' alternative therapists and several thousand therapists not belonging to any organization. Not all these practitioners are medically qualified. I estimate that about 1500 alternative therapists are doctors. Some of these are also general practitioners.

Compared with 46 million contacts between general practitioners and patients, at least 6 million contacts were also made with alternative therapists. One can estimate that in 1979, 7–8% of all those over 18 consulted an alternative therapist, while 60–70% of the total population consulted their general practitioner. Twenty percent of all inhabitants consult an alternative therapist on one or more occasion during their lives.

Alternative therapies in the Netherlands

Our classification of alternative therapies in the Netherlands differs from that in the United Kingdom.

Acupuncture

For several decades acupuncture has been rather popular. About 1600 practitioners are active in this field, the majority in one of the six acupuncture organizations. At least 50% of all therapists are medically qualified — general practitioners, anaesthetists, dentists and others; while 40% are physiotherapists. A very small minority only has received training in one of the four private training courses which are not related to universities or medical schools. Acupuncture is not taught in either undergraduate or in postgraduate medical education. Some doctors practice acupuncture exclusively. However, many doctors and physiotherapists mix acupuncture with their other work.

Homoeopathy

Homoeopathy in the Netherlands is the oldest professionalized alternative therapy. Most homoeopaths operate in the field of primary care. Many of them are GPs with a list of their own, but all homoeopaths can be consulted by patients on the list of a regular GP who prefers a homoeopathic therapy.

Anthroposophical Medicine

The ideas of Rudolf Steiner are becoming increasingly popular in the Netherlands. This results in a subculture, specially in education. Many primary schools are based upon Steiner's ideas and the reputation of anthroposophical care for mentally handicapped children is broadly respected. At the moment there are about 350 anthroposophical general practitioners who provide

101

more or less regular medical care. Their particular philosophy allows them to draw practical lessons from other concepts of illness to give their work a specific flavour.

Chiropractic

In the Netherlands chiropractic is practiced on only a very small scale. However, this does not mean that "chiropractic-like" skills are not popular.

Manual Therapy

Various schools come under the heading of "manual therapy" which includes chiropractic. Osteopathy, in its original form, is practised only by very few. However, at least four schools have developed, based upon ideas drawn from both chiropractic and osteopathy. Besides these schools the orthopaedic medicine developed by Cyriax is popular amongst GPs and physiotherapists. Many professions use this method in their daily work.

Medical Herbalism

Phytotherapy is practiced by very few doctors. Since 1973 several university departments of pharmacology have coordinated research in phytotherapy through a Combined Working Party but, despite this, research is only done on a small scale. Other herbalists base their knowledge upon ancient experience related to folk medicine. In the past, herbalism was one of the most popular therapies outside professional medicine. With the rise of the pharmaceutical industry it declined, but there is now resurgence of interest in herbalism, which stems from the public's increasingly critical attitude toward drugs.

About 30 doctors in the Netherlands practice cellular therapy, advocated by Paul Niehans to stimulate regeneration of tissues and cells. A few others concentrate on parenteral enzyme therapy, hoping to influence the neurohormonal system. One of these enzymes, vasolastine, was said to have a positive effect on arteriosclerosis and many patients instituted legal proceedings in order to obtain reimbursement for this therapy out of medical insurance funds, so far without result.

Natural Therapy

Many procedures come under this heading: hydrotherapy in different forms, dietary therapy of many kinds, bowel cleaning, heliotherapy and many other treatments. In many cases practitioners in this field combine natural therapy with herbalism. Some of them practice iridology, others medical astrology. Finally, to complete the picture, there are about 10 practitioners of Christian Science and faith healing is practiced in different religious situations.

Overlapping practices

These data suggest that at least 5500 persons practice one or more types of alternative therapy, but there are probably many more. Statistics are even less reliable for the estimated number of medical doctors who use alternative therapies, but there are perhaps 1500 of these practitioners in the Netherlands practising chiefly acupuncture, homoeopathy, anthroposophic medicine and to a lesser extent manual therapy.

What then is the relationship between conventional and alternative practices in the Netherlands? General practitioners who practise acupuncture will do so not only for patients on their own list, but also, to a small extent, for other patients. Consultation with specialists is only possible after referral by the GP. Most private insurance companies reimburse for this treatment but the medical insurance fund has not done so to date. There is professional opposition against acupuncture but it is not strong. Younger doctors in particular show little opposition to it. Though many doctors do not take acupuncture seriously, others find it useful for several complaints in which conventional therapy has failed.

Homoeopathy is practiced by those who have their own list of patients. In most cases, they also treat patients who are on the list of an orthodox general practitioner. In addition to these doctors, about 1000 GPs prescribe homoeopathic drugs without adopting the philosophy of the system and in many cases do so at the special request of their patients.

General practitioners involved in anthroposophy usually practice in a city where many anthroposophists are to be found and practice this therapy within the normal medical organization

103

of the Netherlands; for example, they take part in shared night and weekend services.

General practitioners who practise manual therapy use it, in most cases, as part of their normal work. However, a few doctors employ this therapy exclusively. Doctors who practice herbalism, natural therapy or the more peripheral alternative therapies function more or less outside the medical community.

Education and training

Since alternative therapies in the Netherlands are often practised by doctors, training is generally on a part-time basis.

There are three acupuncture courses for doctors and one course for physiotherapists. Most last for 8–10 days each year for three years and are associated with 100–150 hours of clinical practice. An important indication of the change which has taken place in the attitude of orthodox medicine towards acupuncture is that, in the autumn of 1987, the University of Groningen will start a course training in acupuncture, in close cooperation with the Academy for Traditional Chinese Medicine in Shanghai. Two Chinese doctors will cooperate with a Dutch neurologist and a dentist. The Department will provide undergraduate and postgraduate teaching, approved by the Chinese Academy in Shanghai.

Five part-time courses in homoeopathy offer doctors 10 days of instruction a year for two years and others 12 days a year for seven years, though lay persons are not allowed to practice medicine under the existing law. A new law will define the treatment which lay persons in future will be permitted to give. Anthroposophical doctors receive vocational training of one year with 50% of the time spent on theory and 50% on practice. Training in manual therapy is possible in several schools, one of which has a three-year training programme for doctors and physiotherapists, 40 days per year. Another course is more concentrated: three days a week for one year. Many doctors and physiotherapists are trained in the Cyriax method in a course involving 15 days of instruction over 18 months. There is no education in chiropractic and, in most cases, medical herbalism is practiced by laymen. There is one course for doctors, which provides 20 days of teaching annually for four years.

104

The need for registration

If alternative therapies are to have an accepted place in Netherlands medicine, the problem of unqualified therapists will have to be solved and the role fo the Dutch Medical Association will be important. All practicing doctors are registered by the Dutch Medical Association and registration is required for employment in the community and in hospitals. Medical insurance funds and private insurances only remunerate registered doctors. It appears likely that within the next 20 years special registers will be needed for doctors who practice alternative therapies. Existing rules for registration require the completion of approved educational and training programmes which have been subjected to quality control.

There are signs that the Dutch Medical Association is now more open to these ideas. On the other hand, many doctors who use these techniques will hesitate to compromise their standing with their professional organization. When, however, alternative therapies are officially recognized in the Netherlands, it is clear that universities and medical schools which have held aloof from research in this field, will have to play a role.

In the Netherlands, the need for collaboration between conventional and alternative systems of medicine has been recognized. The future will depend upon mutual acceptance and modesty on the part of doctors concerning our own particular record of achievement.

Selected References

Alternatieve geneeswijzen in Nederlands; rapport van de Commissie Alternatieve Geneeswijzen. Staatsuitgeverij: Den Haag, 1981.

Eijk P van. *Geneeswijzen in Nederlands en Vlaanderen*. Seventh edition; Gewijzigde druk. Deventer: Ankh Hermes, 1986.

Maassen van den Brink M H, Vorst H C M. *Beroepsorganisaties Alternatieve Geneeswijzen; een Inventariserend Onderzoek*. University of Amsterdam, Subfaculty of Psychology, 1986.

Statutory Recognition of So-called Associated Health Service Professions. An Anomaly in Medical Politics

Harold C. Gaier
South African Homoeopathic Association
Berea, Durban, South Africa

In South Africa one refers to complementary or alternative therapies as the Associated Health Service Professions. These are distinguished from the Supplementary Health Services Professions, which include physiotherapists, optometrists, pharmacists, podiatrists, psychologists and so on. What I shall describe could be called an anomaly in medical politics. It relates to the statutory recognition of the Associated Health Service Professions by the South African regulatory, governmental bodies.

Nature of the denouement

During December 1974 the Homoeopaths, Naturopaths, Osteopaths and Herbalists Act became effective in the Republic of South Africa.[1] Here began the process of legislative recognition for these disciplines. The fifth of these professions, namely chiropractic, had a similar Act passed separately for itself nearly three years earlier.[2] Only existing College records establishing the prior enrolment of a student and verifiable academic training in his profession(s) would entitle an individual to apply, respectively, for student or practitioner registration, although the majority were then also obliged to submit themselves to stringent examinations in the natural sciences and in their professional subject(s).

The internationally set examinations were also monitored by the South African Department of Health, originally the ultimate registration authority. These were the confidence-building lengths to which the Council of the now recognized Professional Association did, in fact, go to in order to establish the credentials of these disparaged professions in the eyes of both the public

107

and the Ministry of Health. Then followed their "Code of Ethics" necessitating an appropriate amendment to the Act.[3] This amendment gave far-reaching investigative powers to the Professional Association and consequent disciplinary powers to a designated officer of the Department of Health. No new practitioner or student could be registered and no future training might be offered, except for students who were registered at that time. These professions were legislatively predestined to die out.

The Minister of Health now had two choices. The first was incorporation into the South African Medical and Dental Council of these possibly destabilizing, disruptive, therapeutic oddities. Other "adversaries" had been neutralized by amalgamation. The chiropodists joined, and re-emerged as podiatrists, the opticians emerged as optomotrists. The second choice was the creation of an independent statutory Board or Council for these five misfits. With Act 63 of 1982, the Parliament of the Republic of South Africa opted for the latter alternative.[4] The Associated Health Services, through their AHS Professions Board, decided to advance on three fronts.

The first was to hark back on the issues surrounding proper conduct and ethical standards as they ought to pertain to these professions. The result was the model "Code of Ethics", which was copied and adopted in its entirety, almost verbatim, by another profession.

Secondly, the Board promulgated indispensable regulations regarding non-orthodox medicines.

Thirdly the Board requested the Human Sciences Research Council of South Africa to conduct an enquiry on "The Experiences of South Africans relative to Chiropractic and Homoeopathy".[5] The results were astonishing.

They showed that improvements consistently in excess of 80% were achieved in patients who had consistently failed with orthodox medicines. They provided the parliamentarians with the answers to the most controversial two-part question: "Is there a place for these professions and do they satisfy a social need?" The answer, obtained through a thorough, independent survey was a resounding "yes". The way to further legislative progress had now been opened. During June 1985 Parliament approved the 1985 AHS Professions Amendment Act, providing, *inter alia*, for the training and registration of homoeopaths and chiropractors.[6]

The process of maturation

What led up to the 1974 Homoeopaths, Naturopaths, Osteopaths and Herbalists Act? The well-established chiropractors, who could not be swept away after years of practice without grossly offending against Common Law, were placed in a state of suspended animation within their own "terminal Act" in 1971. All other non-orthodox medical professions were, however, destined to be outlawed by the rather stealthily prepared 1974 Medical, Dental and Supplementary Health Services Professions Act, which was to ride roughshod over them.

The herbalists, osteopaths, naturopaths, but particularly the homoeopaths (about 3000 of them in all) orchestrated a protest campaign through their patients. It is said that the then Minister of Health actually received 40,000 telegrams and letters of protest from patients on one particular day. With unseemly haste a so-called "exception Act", modelled upon the Chiropractic Act of three years previously was put together for these four professions, while the orthodox medical establishment was pacified. One would merely have to wait a couple of decades and only orthodox practitioners would be left in the field.

There then followed some remarkably astute moves on the part of the leadership in the non-orthodox camp.

1. The various professional associations joined to form one single Professional Association which was then officially recognized by Parliament as the spokesman for those four professions.

2. Those inadequately trained in the professions were simply refused registration, due to the stringent standards applied by their own single association.

3. The three training colleges in South Africa were closed down at the behest of this same Professional Association itself, which promptly lulled the orthodox medical establishment into a state of complacency and of false security.

4. The Association was successful in getting favourable decisions handed down in the Supreme Court with regard to the appellation "Doctor". The title "Dr" would have to be

109

qualified by *homoeopath* or *osteopath*, etc. and a practitioner might not lead the public to believe that he held a medical qualification, if he, in fact, did not.

5. The Association also succeeded in legally repudiating the Medical and Dental Council's strong disapproval of patient referrals between heterodox and orthodox practitioners, on the grounds that this would be prejudicial to the public's health and would go beyond the scope of the parliamentary enactment.

A little also needs to be said about the other battles that were fought concurrently for the scientific acceptance of the heterodox medical paradigm and the justification for its claim to distinctness. It began with the announcement that we, the heterodox medical establishment, were not opposed to the scientific endeavour but only to the inability of that world view to locate itself properly in a larger context. We steadfastly maintained that there was no way it could be held that, in medicine at least, the orthodox tenets were more scientifically rational than ours. The rebuttal was foreseeable: "Where are those supportive experiments, which are both repeatable and have yielded statistically significant results?" The Professional Association succeeded in obtaining the opportunity in 1981 to present its scientific evidence in a very condensed form to the South African Medical and Dental Council. We choose the case for homoeopathy.

Is homoeopathy anti-scientific? we asked. Since 1928, a series of biological, chemical and physical experiments have uniformly demonstrated the existence of some physico-chemical force in homoeopathy's molecular dilutions. However, these experiments over more than half a century are dispersed geographically and the spread of scientific evidence has been too sparse to have had a noticeable effect.

At the end of this presentation, the gentlemen from the Medical and Dental Council seemed to be asleep. That signalled to the Minister that there was no hope of ever accommodating these heresies in mainstream medicine. He had no alternative but to report to Parliament that the South African Medical and Dental Council had manifestly set itself against the incorporation of these apocryphal medical disciplines. But then Parliament was prepared for this.

An uneasy truce between incongruous competitors

The Cinderella status of the five AHS Professions has vanished. Virtually all Medical Aid Schemes in South Africa (these are privately run and almost all breadwinners are voluntary contributors) pay for the services and medications of non-orthodox practitioners. Many pharmacists have taken a simple supplementary course to familiarize themselves with the medicinal principles associated with the rudiments of heterodox pharmacy.

Perhaps the most telling compliment was inadvertently paid to the AHS Professions recently by the Secretary of the South African Pharmacy Association. He reproved his own profession's inability to assert themselves effectively and he highlighted the contrasting, rapid accomplishments of the numerically much weaker but far more single-minded AHS Professions in this respect.

The degree to which heterodoxy has drawn level with orthodoxy can be judged from the minimum standards set for the six-year full-time academic training course for practitioners.

1st Year: Anatomy I, Biology, Chemistry, Physics, Basic Philosophy.

2nd Year: Anatomy II, Biochemistry, Community Health, Pathology I, Physiology, Epidemiology, Microbiology, Psychology, Sociology.

3rd Year: Diagnostics I, Emergency Medicine, Jurisprudence, Materia Medica I, Pathology II, Practice Management, Psychiatry.

4th Year: Clinical Homoeopathy I, Diagnostics II, Homoeo-pharmaceutics, Materia Medica II.

5th Year: Clinical Homoeopathy II, Materia Medica III, Research Methodology.

6th Year: Internship.

Within Clinical Homoeopathy have been included all aspects of naturopathy, whereas herbalism has been included in Materia Medica teaching as well as in homoeopharmaceutics. Chiropractors will do the same first two years and start branching towards the manipulative therapies in years 3–5, with an internship directed towards chiropractic, which includes

111

osteopathy. Each year is comprised of a minimum of 1000 hours of study spread over 36 weeks, thus ensuring 28 hours of lectures and practicals per week. The student will be expected to put in additional study time of at least 20 to 30 hours per week.

The intention is to produce a graduate who can fill a meaningful role in the South African Health Care Delivery System, to the benefit of all population groups and one who will be fully integrated into the small Community Health Care Centres that are destined to replace the mammoth hospitals in providing primary health delivery of the future.

If we in South Africa (where stubbornness has been refined to a degree of excellence unsurpassed elsewhere) can do it, so can others.

References

1 RSA Act No. 52 of 1974: Homoeopaths, Naturopaths, Osteopaths and Herbalists Act, 1974.
2 RSA Act No. 76 of 1971: Chiropractors Act, 1971.
3 RSA Act No. 40 of 1980: Homoeopaths, Naturopaths, Osteopaths and Herbalists Amendment Act, 1980.
4 RSA Act No. 63 of 1982: Associated Health Service Professions Act, 1982.
5 Steenekamp C S. South Africans' Experience of Chiropractic and Homoeopathy. Research Finding OSC-1/1985. Centre for Social Research Data, Human Sciences Research Council, Pretoria.
6 RSA Act No. 108 of 1985: Associated Health Service Professions Amendment Act, 1985.

Clinical, Academic and Socio-Political Collaboration in the United States

Robert M. Duggan
*Traditional Acupuncture Institute, Columbia,
Maryland 21044, USA*

As a clinician, teacher and acupuncturist, I will use the experience of our profession to illustrate some issues of concern in regard to the practice of complementary and alternative medicine in the United States.

I will touch on issues of research, clinical practice and social policy in the particular context of the USA. However, we have much to learn from the experience of the United Kingdom. You have a Council for Complementary and Alternative Medicine. You have a Research Council for Complementary Medicine which publishes a journal and looks at methodological questions. There is also a proposed Centre for Complementary Health Studies at Exeter University, something that we are beginning to talk about in Maryland, but no similar institution exists in the USA. I note that the *Lancet*[1] has recently published a report of studies on acupuncture and homoeopathy. I cannot yet imagine similar reports in the *New England Journal of Medicine*.

A period of change

Our situation is very different from that described by Professor van Es in Holland and Dr Gaier in South Africa. I envy their ability to speak of one unified legislative process. In the USA, legislation and regulation on issues of health are carried out at State level, so this process goes on in 50 distinct jurisdictions. Thus we have 50 distinct models from which to learn. I will try to generalize and I will begin with my own experience in Maryland.

In the Maryland Legislature when the issue of the regulation of acupuncture arose there were two possible starting points. One was negotiation between professions (doctors and

113

acupuncturists) on matters of economic competition. On that issue the legislature had little patience. They opposed such discussions. It was clear that they were concerned with the issue of what benefitted the patient. They wanted to hear patients' testimony. They wanted to learn about results based on clinical experience. They wanted to know what assisted healing, and they wanted regulation, not for economic benefit, but as the result of concern for public service.

The end-point is largely dependent on the starting-point. Our experience in the USA is one of amazing change in the public demand for service. In the State of Maryland 10 years ago there were seven acupuncturists who were unlicensed and unregistered, working with physicians. Now there are 140 licensed and registered in the State. We have established criteria for their licensing and registration. They work in a specific collaborative relationship with physicians. Our school graduates approximately 15 students who remain in the State each year. Many practitioners in Maryland have a waiting list. I work in a group practice associated with the school. Last year there were 10,000 treatments in that one clinic alone and 68% of those treatments were covered by various forms of health insurance.

Issues of health

In the US the public is, at the moment, obsessed with issues of health, nutrition and exercise. Colin Greer of the New World Foundation indicated in the *Journal of Traditional Acupuncture*[2] that self-responsibility in health may be one of the few areas in which individuals can maintain a sense of self-control and have a sense of power. The Secretary of Health of the State of Maryland said two years ago that ''In our urge to take technology to its limits we have created a sick-care system rather than a health-care system. Consumers and physicians depend on treatment rather than investing in health. People have become dependent on medicine rather than on themselves. We must turn this around and we must test the alternatives.'' I recall that when we moved to the State of Maryland 12 years ago, we received a letter from that same Health Department saying that what we were doing was illegal.

There has been an enormous change in the public context. That change is furthered by the fact that an increasing percentage of our gross national product is going into health issues. Because of uncontrollable insurance costs, large corporations are seeking ways to control the health care percentage of their budgets. They are studying how to increase the health of their workers and to lower the costs of illness. The Chrysler Corporation discovered that, next to steel, the health of the worker was the second most expensive item in a car's costs. There is both an enormous effort to cut health costs, and a backlash of anger by physicians because of the expectations that have been demanded of them. Again quoting from the Secretary of Health of the State of Maryland: ''Society has great expectations of physicians to know everything, and they often ask them to do things that they are not trained to do.''

The Life Insurance Council of America, which is the trade organization of the major life insurance groups, has produced a projection of health care in the USA for the year 2030. They provide three alternative scenarios, in one of which there are hardly any human beings involved. In another, they project that there will be fewer doctors, very few hospitals and most people will be taking care of themselves in programmes of self-responsibility and community care. They specifically mention the increased use of medicinal herbs, acupuncture, osteopathy, chiropractic and homoeopathy.[3]

Subtle energies

We must also look within the context of what is going on in medicine itself. Dr Robert Becker of the University of Rochester Medical School has recently published a book called *The Body Electric*. Dr Bjorn Norenstrom, who was a member of the Nobel prize committee in Sweden, has published a work on the electrical system of the body and the treatment of tumours with electricity. I noticed recently his presence at a conference in Los Angeles linking his research with that of acupuncturists using the electrical properties of the meridian points.

A study at Stanford University teamed an anaesthesiologist and a surgeon to investigate orthopaedic spinal surgery where there is a large loss of blood. Their controlled studies showed

115

that if the anaesthesiologist made the suggestion that the blood would flow away from the area of surgery, the blood loss was half that compared to the cases where the suggestion was not made.[4] What I am suggesting is that there is a great need for research in what might be called the subtle energies in the body, energies which are associated with herbology, homoeopathy, acupuncture, osteopathy and chiropractic.

Delivering complementary medicine

The words "complementary" and "alternative" are not often used in the USA, perhaps because all systems are free of Federal Government regulation. Osteopathy and chiropractic are large established professions. They have four-year, post-graduate programmes and thousands of practitioners. The Chiropractic Association in recent years has won anti-trust law suits against the established allopathic professions. The amount of suppression has decreased during the past years and the interaction between the osteopathic, chiropractic and allopathic professions is increasing. I should also say that both of these professions, in their efforts to become part of the mainstream, have lost some of their own integrity. For example, in many osteopathic schools in the USA, manipulation is an optional course. Osteopathic graduates are equivalent to allopathic physicians. I mention this because it is an extremely important issue if we are to look at the value which complementary medical traditions bring to patient care. Each has a unique contribution to make and if they are judged by existing standards, that contribution cannot be made. The chiropractic and osteopathic professions in the USA are now in the process of rediscovering their roots.

So many members of Congress were homoeopaths that when the Food and Drug Administration came into existence and laws were passed regarding the development of drugs, these members of Congress were able to protect the existing homoeopathic pharmacopoea. However, the homoeopathic profession decreased greatly in numbers because of a classical union struggle at the turn of the century. It is now beginning to regroup. Training programmes are beginning to develop and it has the remnants of legislation and protection. Many of our State

Legislatures have what we call "sunset " laws, where regulations regarding various professions automatically go out of existence after so many years unless it can be shown that there is a continuing need for them. This year, in the State of Arizona, the homoeopathic regulations were due to lapse and the recommendation from the medical establishment was that they be allowed to do so. The Legislature overruled that recommendation and gave that Board a new tenure. Medical herbalism is a growing interest in the USA, due to interest in Chinese medicine and the introduction of Chinese herbalism and related studies.

The example of acupuncture

There are approximately 5000 licensed acupuncturists in the USA and 25 of the 50 States have established various regulatory mechanisms for that practice. There are 12 state-approved schools and probably more in the process of developing adequate curricula. The State of Maryland allows acupuncture to be practised under medical supervision. Medical advisers to the Legislature had feared that acupuncture, like other complementary therapies, might mask symptoms. However, the State Legislature held that as long as there was protection against that possibility, it saw no reason to prohibit the practice of alternative therapies. In fact, throughout the USA, that protection is provided by prior medical examination and, in consequence, acupuncture has taken a great step forward.

The distinction between allopathic medicine, dealing primarily with organic pathology, and the complementary professions which aim to prevent illness reaching that point, has been one of the main concerns of our Legislatures. Another relates to competence to practice and the protection of the public from charlatans.

In Maryland, we have worked hard at developing cooperation with the medical profession. During the past 10 years we have progressed to the point where I am just about to be afforded facilities at the local hospital following a period in which we have been seen as working together with the local physicians. This has involved establishing mutually agreed procedures acceptable to the hospital authorities, physicians, therapists and patients.

117

There have been clinical benefits. For example, side-effects from radiation therapy have been greatly reduced by the simultaneous use of acupuncture, and complementary therapists have found a role in the management of impending cardiac crises.

The need for research

To demand of a complementary therapy that it should provide all research and clinical amenities to be found in a conventional medical establishment would be quite unrealistic. However, we are making progress. In Maryland, the next stage will involve interactive processes with medical schools. There are programmes at Boston's Beth Israel Hospital which is associated with Harvard Medical School. The Montefiore Hospital in New York has both a clinical programme and a school for ''other therapies'' and Down State Medical Center in New York is using acupuncture for AIDS and drug addiction.

An example of the impact this is having on our culture may be found in Santa Cruz, California, where teachers have discovered that acupressure points are so effective in relaxing children in school that they adapted this technique for slow learners with improvement in the learning ability of those students. This school district now trains 10,000 teachers from all over the USA in the use of these techniques.[5] As a result of research into the effects of acupuncture carried out in 1973, the University of Los Angeles demonstrated that acupuncture has an efficacy beyond that of the placebo response. In January 1986, the journal *Pain*[6] published a comprehensive review of research in acupuncture, taken mainly from the American literature, but made the point that, because no attention had been paid to the qualifications of acupuncturists, reports could not be critically evaluated.

The best review of the literature on acupuncture is that of the physician David Eisenberg, who was the first Fulbright Fellow to be sent to China specifically to investigate Oriental medicine. His book, *Encounters with Chi*[7], is the result. The National Institutes of Health have recently published a report on chronic pain in which, for the first time, acupuncture and the alternative therapies are recommended options for physicians.[8] The American College of Traditional Chinese Medicine in

118

San Francisco has cooperated with the University of San Francisco and with the Botanical Garden of that city to conduct research on the pharmacology of Chinese medical herbs and the Department of Behavioral Medicine at Boston's Beth Israel Hospital is involved in a similar programme in China.

Accreditation and certification

Acupuncture in the USA is now a profession with legally established criteria, due largely to efforts on the part of the acupuncture community itself. It was not the result of Government initiatives and we have followed the system for the accreditation of all other graduate education programmes in the USA. Each school reviews its own curriculum, sets its own goals and standards and monitors student performance. An external team of visitors, which includes both members of the profession and general educators, then makes an on-site visit. That process is monitored at Federal level by an independent council of post-secondary schools acting as an Accreditation Commission whose standards are reviewed by an independent agency.

The most difficult part of the process was to agree common standards and it was considered desirable to attain the equivalent of a Master's Degree, usually involving a five-year period of study after high-school. In fact, most complementary therapy qualifications already require at least a three-year post-college programme and this has been retained as the minimum require-ment for full-time study based on a standard core curriculum. Once uniformity had been achieved, it became easier for acupuncture schools to win approval from State legislators, regulatory bodies and State Departments of Education.

Certification is the criterion of ability to practise, and the acupuncture profession defined the parameters to be measured. Thirty practitioners were asked what skills were essential to practise. The criteria they established were then field-tested by 300 practising acupuncturists and formed the basis for an annual national examination currently being taken by more than 400 candidates. Every State which has adopted this procedure has granted ''grandfathering'' to those who have been practising for five years or more, but all new practitioners must graduate by examination.

119

Further progress depends upon unity within the profession and between the complementary professions. Cooperation, persistence and a willingness to answer every question has been characteristic of the development of acupuncture, osteopathy and chiropractic in the United States. A similar process for herbalism and homoeopathy will be required.

Acknowledgement

The Institute for the Advancement of Health in New York City is a valuable source for the latest research information and I am grateful for the assistance of its President, Miss Eileen Growald Rockefeller, in presenting this paper. Literature on the legislative processes is now available from the Traditional Acupuncture Foundation, American City Building (100), Columbia, Maryland 21044, USA.

References

1 Jobst K, Chen J H, McPherson K, Arrowsmith J, Brown V, Efthimiou J, Fletcher H J, Maciocia G, Mole P, Shifrin K, Lane D J. Controlled trial of acupuncture for disabling breathlessness. *Lancet* 1986; **2**: 1416–9.
2 Greer C. Notes toward an empowering perspective. *Journal of Traditional Acupuncture*, 1985; 33.
3 Life Insurance Council Trend Analysis Program. American Council of Life Insurance, 1850 K Street, N. W., Washington, DC 2006.
4 Bennett H L, Benson D R, Sargo S H. Preoperative suggestions for significantly reduced blood loss during orthopaedic spinal surgery. Paper presented to the American Psychological Association, Los Angeles, August 1985.
5 Physical Response Educational Systems. Santa Cruz County Office of Education, 809-H Bay Avenue, Capitola, CA 95010.
6 Vincent C A, Richardson P H. The evaluation of therapeutic acupuncture: concepts and methods. *Pain* 1986; **24**: 1–40.
7 Eisenberg D. *Encounters with Chi: Exploring Chinese Medicine*. New York: Norton, 1985.
8 National Institutes of Health, Consensus Development Conference Statement: *The Integrated Approach to the Management of Pain*. Bethesda 1986; 11.

International Collaboration
Highlights from the Discussions

Learning from other countries

Professor van Es said that legislation in Holland would still take some years to complete. However, by that time, everyone would have a legal right to treat patients except by specific medical, surgical and obstetric methods and except for the prescribing of specified drugs. The major remaining problem would be one of remuneration. Some therapists would prefer to remain outside the State system. The recommendations of the Commission would not necessarily be adopted by Parliament but if Parliament did not take note of alternative practices, this could lead to serious problems.

Mr Copeland Griffiths contrasted the rudimentary training of Dutch doctors in manipulation with the four-year, full-time course demanded of Dutch chiropractors and Professor van Es explained that many non-medical therapists were at a serious disadvantage because medically qualified practitioners, with little training in chiropractic, were practising it. This posed a threatening situation for non-academic alternative therapists.

Dr Stott wondered to what extent tribal medicine had been integrated with white alternative medicine in South Africa and Mr Gaier explained that a third set of legislative guarantees existed for tribal medicine with laws going back to 1948.

Mr Breen asked about academic requirements for those entering a six-year course of training in alternative medicine and learned from Mr Gaier that, as for any other academic discipline, matriculation was mandatory. In reply to Dr Christie, who asked what alternative training would cost the student, Mr Gaier considered it would be of the same order as that of a conventional medical training.

Again, in relation to South Africa, Dr Wetzler asked whether there was a fringe element and, if so, how it had been dealt with. Mr Gaier explained that there was a community of such therapists, several of whom had arrived from Europe. They were

121

reflexologists and others who could not be registered. There was also a serious anomaly in relation to acupuncturists, since the law did not recognize acupuncture as a separate discipline. It was a problem still awaiting a solution.

Mr Hutchinson was concerned to hear about the dangers of interaction between certain complementary therapies and practitioners of allopathic medicine in America, which had resulted in some colleagues no longer teaching manipulation, but he reported that the chiropractic and osteopathic professions in the States were aware of this problem and were taking steps to rectify it.

Dr Patterson reported an important example of increasing informational cooperation in his field of work. First, a data bank in musculoskeletal medicine had been set up in Zurich. Secondly, the International Federation of Manual Medicine would be holding its next triennial congress in London in 1989, when a substantial part of one of the four days of the programme would be devoted to the contributions of complementary medicine. Thirdly, for the first time, there would be a meeting at which three different groups of people with interests in musculoskeletal medicine would be getting together for discussions, not only between themselves, but also at a joint symposium with the Institute of Orthopaedic Medicine, the London College of Osteopathic Medicine and the British Association of Manipulative Medicine.

The benefits of collaboration in Britain were underlined by Dr Peter Nixon, who drew upon his own experience in the Cardiac Department of Charing Cross Hospital to illustrate how the best of modern technology could be united with the best of human healing skills in an integrated effort on behalf of the patient. Such teamwork created a mutual desire to see the patient succeed and to provide support when problems arose. The integrating role of the occupational therapist should be recognized.

An optimistic future for collaboration?

Lord Kindersley said that it was unfortunate that the very sensible recommendations made by the Dutch Commission had not yet been accepted by the Dutch Parliament. It seemed likely

122

that doctors with a part-time training in natural therapies would have a preferred position over therapists with a full four-year training course behind them. Instead of the Dutch providing us with a model to emulate, they were perhaps giving us warnings of the pitfalls to avoid.

By contrast, the South Africans had produced an appropriate model but only after a bitter struggle. He hoped that the same sort of confrontation would not be necessary in Britain to achieve the same objective. He thought that the very existence of these Colloquia showed that the ends could be achieved by gentler means. Certainly he was impressed by the very comprehensive training programmes developed in South Africa.

British participants should be grateful that they did not have to deal with 50 independently minded States, as was the case in the United States of America. Britain did however belong to the United States of Europe and the Dutch experience made it even more important that we should establish a sensible model to be used within the European context. He had been interested in Mr Duggan's account of the successful anti-trust actions which had been taken by the Chiropractors' Association against the medical establishment. He had also been intrigued by the loss of integrity of practitioners once they had become established.

To turn to the position in the United Kingdom, he had not been surprised when the BMA issued a Report which was generally critical of natural therapy. Interestingly enough, however, this Report did not seem to reflect the views of its membership. There was a natural resistance to the unorthodox by the orthodox in any profession and he understood that Pasteur and Freud had both been opposed, in their time, for this reason. The *Which* surveys found that one in seven of their 28,000 members said that they had used some form of complementary or alternative medicine during the previous 12 months. If this reflected the national situation then eight million people in the UK were using such medicine during 1985. These figures were crude, but they were clear enough to show that it was high time to ensure that standards within these therapies were adequate and regulated by some body equivalent to the General Medical Council.

The therapy organizations themselves were well aware of this need. The General Council and Register of Osteopaths and the British Chiropractic Association had tabled a Bill which would allow standards to be set and regulated. It seemed that the traditional route to self-validation was being followed, with the Government adding its blessing, if somewhat reluctantly.

They had heard that considerable advances were being made in research, in clinical collaboration and in the understanding of the socio-political issues. First and foremost was the understanding between doctors and therapists; the raising of standards; the establishment of parameters for research; draft legislation for the regulation of therapeutic practices and acceptance that complementary medicine was an area with which orthodox doctors must concern themselves. Last but not least was the growing interest of the public, without which none of these changes would have occurred as quickly as they had. The Colloquia had showed what other countries were doing, and had demonstrated that orthodox and unorthodox practitioners could find some common ground. He had been particularly impressed by the results of the South African chiropractic and homoeopathic studies and believed that the ethical code, which had been established there for the complementary therapies, would repay careful study.

Failing to learn from history

Sir James Watt felt that international collaboration had provided a rewarding theme for the final Colloquium. Lord Kindersley had rightly pointed out the opposition which even conventional practitioners have encountered in the advancement of medical knowledge, mentioning particularly Freud and Pasteur. Equally, Lord Lister who saw the implications of Pasteur's work and introduced antiseptic surgery, was vigorously attacked by his colleagues when he came to London.

However, in the Twentieth Century, some are just beginning to allow an alternative point of view, and there is now international evidence of cautious acceptance of some complementary techniques. Although the BMA report acknowledged that the discovery of endorphins provided a rational explanation for the success of acupuncture, it found it necessary to issue a warning. Others, less critical, believe that acupuncture, because it is explicable, can now be practised. The question then arose whether effective therapeutic measures should be withheld until such time as medical scientists find an acceptable rationale — for that would invalidate much conventional prescribing, as well as that of, say, homoeopathy.

The history of scurvy in the hands of orthodox physicians is very instructive. Despite the fact that for hundreds of years, empirical observations indicated that oranges and lemons prevented and cured scurvy, the various influences upon scientific thinking over the centuries diverted attention from this simple observation and condemned thousands of seamen to death.

Surgeons were no better. In the Sixteenth Century, William Clowes, a surgeon at St Bartholomew's Hospital, learned empirically how to treat burns almost as effectively as we do today, choosing plant remedies relevant to the depth of the injury and the stage of treatment. But it has taken us 400 years to recognize that those plant remedies actually contained the various active ingredients which were essential to the treatment. Some contained tannins which provided a protective covering, others contained antibiotics, and others provided enzymatic debridement of the slough. Clowes recognized too that these patients required fluid replacement, which he provided by boiled water. This was in the Sixteenth Century, yet the history of orthodox therapy reveals that, in the Eighteenth Century, burns were being treated with lead lotions which led to death from toxic absorption. That lesson was never learned. In the First World War, picric acid of even greater toxicity was used, and in the Second World War, the use of tannic acid led to liver damage.

There is therefore a danger in saying that ''until I have an explanation which accords with current scientific thinking, I am unable to accept the remedy''. Perhaps, then, these Colloquia have been able to bring a little enlightenment to our orthodox colleagues. They have also brought enlightenment to our complementary colleagues, who no longer regard orthodox practitioners with suspicion.

History provides yet another cautionary tale. We have learnt from the American experience that recognition of some therapies led to autonomy which induced complacency. Lord Lister did more than anyone else to make the techniques of modern surgery possible and, in consequence, became the benefactor of millions of patients. Yet, when he became President of the Royal Society, he had become so obsessed by the problems of bacterial contamination that he attributed the cause of scurvy to ''ptomaine poisoning''.

That was in 1900, and as a result of such seemingly authoritative pronouncements, Scott took no antiscorbutics to the South Pole in 1911. His party perished because he believed that sterilized foods rather than vitamin-rich foods would avoid nutritional problems. Perhaps our complementary friends will take note because there is a real danger that once our views are accepted, we can become blind to the contributions of others in different fields.

The Public View

How do the public see the current discussion between orthodox and conventional therapy? The lay person's view is compared with that of a member of the Christian Healing Ministry, both "outsiders" to the central debate, but both with valuable perspectives to contribute.

Christopher Hamel-Cooke comments on the way that the social case-worker may have usurped the pastoral role of the priest. However, Christian counselling has a special value of its own in helping the client to choose one of the various alternatives open to him. Ideally too, such counselling is as "non-judgemental" as any from a lay practitioner, though it does concentrate more on the client's ultimate purpose in life.

Katharine Whitehorn left the Colloquia convinced that the basic distinction between the orthodox and the complementary had to do with the different theoretical models held by each. However, she suggests that both groups should follow the truly "scientific" principle of first establishing what effects their treatments actually produce, then discussing the how and why. By that means they may reach a level of agreement which will inevitably be to the patient's benefit.

The Ingredients of Christian Counselling*

Christopher K. Hamel-Cooke
Marylebone Christian Counselling Centre, London NW1 5LT

Among the many divisions occasioned by the growing apart of the medical and clerical professions is that between Counselling and Pastoralia. The clergy of the Church have always been expected to be pastors to their people. The distinguishing mark of the bishop is his shepherd's crook. His ministry is modelled upon the image of Christ, the Good Shepherd. In the confessional, the penitent seeks not only penance and absolution, but also counsel and advice. Where the formality of the confessional is not the norm, the relationship of the priest or minister to his people has always been seen in terms of pastoral care—indeed he often speaks of his people as ''his flock''. He does not of course think of them only collectively. A shepherd knows each of his sheep ''by name''.

Rise of the case-worker

Alongside the ministry of the Church, the medical profession has developed its own ancillary in what is usually called case-work. With the insights learned from the study of psychology and sociology, case-workers and counsellors have become professionals in their own right and have often made the pastoral care of the clergy seem amateur.

As the rift between doctor and priest is healed, so the insights of the social worker become more readily available to the priest. Nor is the traffic only in one direction. Each has something to learn from the other. The rapport may begin with the learning of each other's language and the understanding of each other's basic concepts.

The furtherance of this coming together has been greatly helped by the work of the Institute of Religion and Medicine. Founded

---

* Reprinted from *Health is for God*. London: Arthur James, 1986 with kind permission.

by Michael Ramsey, when Archbishop of Canterbury, it brings doctors and clergy together with their ancillary colleagues in local field groups, to share each other's concerns. It also works at a more academic level. In recent years doctors and clergy have studied and written about the common ground between them and explored in some depth the interface between religion and medicine. A major contribution of the late Dr Lambourne, psychiatrist and theologian, was the founding of the Diploma in Pastoral Studies at Birmingham University, where students from both the medical and theological disciplines come together in pursuit of this end.

Despite the undoubted progress and the joy that the drift is in the right direction, it has to be acknowledged that there is a great discrepancy of skill and capacity in both the medical and clerical professions. Some doctors and some priests are virtually without counselling skills, would make no pretence to have them, may even despise them—yet despite this limitation may remain in other respects good doctors and good priests.

The medical profession has however at its disposal, in hospital and in general practice, the assistance, when the doctor needs to call upon it, of the trained social worker. The clergy are less organized. They recognize their need to be available to give help and pastoral care to the individual members of their flock. Some few have dedicated their whole life's ministry to the direction of souls and have brought not only healing but holiness too, to those who have turned to them for help. Others have sought to improve their pastoral skills by benefitting from the insights of the other professions and undergoing in-service training or sabbatical post-graduate study. In consequence, some clergy are thought of as ''Christian counsellors'' and some churches as agencies of this ministry.

Secular and Christian counselling

It may be asked, what expectation of difference would there by between a secular counsellor and a specifically Christian one? The Christian counsellor must not be less professional than his secular counterpart. He ought to be expected to have all that the other has, and more too. The ''more'' will not only be an added dimension but an enhancement of all the others. Let us examine this further by looking at some of the basic principles of counselling, and seeing in what way the Christian faith of the counsellor makes this difference.

The counsellor is taught the importance of "acceptance". He learns that, as a principle of action, he must deal with this client as he really is. This does not of course mean approval, but it does mean acknowledging the reality of the situation and accepting the client accordingly. He knows that if the client is or feels rejected—and he may come expecting and even inviting that reaction—that will at best add to the client's malaise and at worst result in the breakdown of the relationship almost as soon as it has begun.

The Christian counsellor accepts all this. But he also perceives that his client is a fellow human being, made like himself, in the image of God. His worth, his value, is inalienable and the counsellor perceives his value as an agent of healing and a means of restoring the distorted image of the human nature which is also divine. The case-worker thus has to make himself acceptable to his client as a step in making the client acceptable to himself. He does so because he knows that God accepts all His children just as they are and that common fatherhood makes all men his brethren.

He also remembers that our Lord accepted the most rejected people in the society to which he came—befriended them, suffered because of His concern for them.

A host of difficulties

There are of course, for the secular counsellor and for the Christian, many difficulties; in all of them the Christian is assisted by his faith and commitment. First, the counsellor must recognize as an obstacle the non-acceptance of something in himself. The Christian knows that though he must seek to come to terms with this, God already accepts him. He is then helped to accept the unacceptable in others.

The counsellor knows the danger of imputing to the client his own feelings and so assuming that he actually knows how the client is feeling. The Christian perception of the absolute uniqueness of every human being helps him to guard against this.

131

The counsellor is aware that he like all men may be guilty of bias and prejudice. The Christian often starts in his client's eyes at a disadvantage because he may be assumed to have such prejudice! It is sadly true that many people have distorted ideas of the convictions upon which Christian work is based and assume them to be or likely to lead to prejudice. No doubt, too, they often are and do. But the faith of the Christian ought to be an antidote to bias. His creed should help him to know and understand the creeds of others. His culture he knows to be one among many that God has created. He therefore respects his client even against the client's rejection of himself, whichever his background and encumbrances may be. He treats him as a unique individual. He knows him "by name", as God knows all His children by name. He will show it by using it.

Acceptance carries with it an attitude to the client which must never be seen as judgemental. The secular counsellor knows this. He is not there to determine guilt or innocence; he is there to identify need. The Victorian concept of the "deserving poor" has no place in his vocabulary. Worthiness is irrelevant. He is there to help not to punish or to blame, nor indeed to praise! He knows how often his client will have come from an environment in which he may have received moral criticism. He also knows that the client's gross failure to live by the standard and norms of society does not necessarily mean that he does not accept or value these standards. Often he longs to have them reinforced and seeks help to enable him to live up to them.

The Christian counsellor adds to these perceptions his knowledge that "God's power is shown chiefly in mercy and pity." He knows that there is a sense in which God is our judge. He knows also that there is no sense in which he is. He knows that God's judgement is not vindictive but reaches out to achieve the reconciliation of those who err. He knows that despite the seeming evidence to the contrary, that God is a God of love and compassion. He knows that all Christians are called by the fact of their discipleship to exercise those graces—and none more so than those who are called to serve in the rightly-called caring professions.

Helping the client to choose

It is important to lay hold upon the nature of God's judgement upon which the Christian Ethic is based. I once had an interesting dispute with a secular social worker. He was a Marriage Guidance Counsellor and after a lecture on the work of that excellent organization, he was asked, "Does the counsellor ever moralize?" An immediate and emphatic, "No" greeted the question. But then he added, "Of course, the counsellor may observe upon the logical consequences of the choices that people make." He was taken aback when asked what he thought was the difference between that and moralizing. Strictly speaking there is none. A Christian moralizes, or explains the Christian Ethic solely in terms of consequence! Judgement, properly understood, is the logical consequence of the choices we make. So the Christian counsellor does not himself judge. He knows that he too is under judgement — having to live with the consequence of the exercise of his own free will.

The counsellor is taught the importance of client self-determination. It was Oscar Wilde who observed that though bad advice is always bad, good advice is absolutely disastrous! It robs the client of his capacity for making his own decisions, of accepting responsibility for his own life. The Christian counsellor can go on to say that everyman is made in the image of God, that his freedom of choice is his most God-like possession; he can show how God longs to renew that image in him and to restore to him the supreme dignity of being human. His advice as a counsellor will only be to draw the attention of his client to the saving words and works of Christ and help him then to work out his own healing and salvation.

The Christian recognizes that just as God does not destroy an individual's right to go his own way, however deleterious that way may appear to be, so he must resist any temptation to take charge of his client for his own good, to persuade him against his own judgement or to manipulate him or his situation to bring about what he, rather than the client, thinks should happen.

The counsellor is taught to beware of his own emotional involvement. If he has no compassion, he will be useless to his client. If he becomes over involved, he will quickly forfeit his capacity to help. He knows that what his client presents to him

133

will be both *facts* and *feelings*. Everyone's problem is the sum of the objective reality and the subjective thoughts and feelings about that reality. Even if the objective reality is not a reality but something entirely imaginary, the subjective response remains the same and in itself entirely real. The case-worker seeks to make an appropriate response both to the facts and to the feelings about them. He tries to express that response only in so far as the expression will help his client to know and achieve his purposes. The Christian counsellor seeks to interpret the facts in a way consonant with God's activity in human history. What is God saying in this situation?

Compassion and confidentiality

He also exercises the compassion of Christ and shows his own, as part of that fellowship in Christ's own sufferings in which both he and his client share. He does not therefore bear the client's suffering alone; he does so in fellowship and partnership with his Lord. He seeks to help his client to do the same. He will help the client to express his feelings to the degree which is appropriate, not only to himself but also to God.

The anger and the bitterness and the hostility which may overcome the client and may at times need to find an outlet, the counsellor must be ready to accept. But the Christian counsellor will help him to direct his feelings however hostile to God Himself. He will show that God is the source of all comfort, that His shoulders are broad enough to accept and His heart wide enough to forgive all the hostility in the world.

The counsellor is taught to be confidential. He must be trusted with the confidences of the client. The Christian counsellor knows that God Himself is privy to all that has been exchanged and bind the confidences with the seal of the confessional—to betray the client is to betray Christ Himself.

Fit for God

The counsellor has the temporal welfare of his client as his first consideration. He seeks to enable the client to return to his environment and then to live with a sufficient degree of usefulness and contentment. The Christian counsellor has that end in view too; but he asks a more ultimate question. To what

134

purpose his temporal welfare? Is not this life a journey? How can a man be fit if he does not know what he is fit for? So he must seek to be fit for God and His glory. Fit to be a useful member of society. Yes, to be happy and content within himself; but also to be fit for God, fit for the advancement of His Kingdom. A man who has no sense of his ultimate purpose and destiny is not, in the Christian sense, well at all.

So the Christian counsellor not only adds God to the relationship of his client; he sees God in all the others and interprets them accordingly. It will be as natural and normal for him to pray with and for his client as it is to talk to Him himself. This does not of course mean that he will always do so. The client may have no such desire, may be angry or embarrassed by the suggestion. The Christian counsellor must ever seek to be sensitive to what at any given moment, with any particular person, is apt and appropriate and so his Christian faith and conviction must only become explicit when it will help the client for them to do so.

A Lay-person's View of the Colloquia

Katharine Whitehorn
*Open Section, Royal Society of Medicine,
London W1M 8AE, UK*

There is one respect in which almost all ordinary people are different from almost all doctors. For the latter, there is a clear distinction between the medicine which they have learned, and the realms which lie outside. They know what is medicine and what isn't. The layman starts from quite a different position. All the way from someone's cool hand on a headache, through childhood Elastoplast and laxatives, aspirin and Aunt Nellie's brimstone mixture, to what the chemist says, what the nurse and the GP and the hospital consultant say, there is, for us, a continuous and cloudy spectrum, instantly mixed with vague feelings of well-being, languor, exhilaration, the dumps.

It is this generalised perception that causes the layman to be credulous and ignorant, from one viewpoint; or open-minded, from another. We are not scientists, yet we have to believe in science; we cannot ourselves follow the experiments, assess the validity of this treatment or that; we have to take *everything* on trust except our own immediate experience. So whom should we trust?

Professional mistakes

Contrary to what some orthodox medical practitioners think (or perhaps only say), it is by no means certain that even a clear diagnosis, let alone a perfect cure, can be expected whenever you go to the doctor. As a journalist, and through the Patient's Association, I doubtless hear about more than my fair share of professional mistakes; but every family has its tale to tell.

My best friend died of diabetes, undiagnosed for six months because his GP sent him to a leg man for his sore leg, and no-one did any tests. My sister-in-law has been hospitalized three times for iatrogenic disorders. A retired policeman of my

137

acquaintance, tired of being told of the harm that can be done by osteopathy, counted up how many of his own friends had had their backs made better by osteopaths, how many worse. The score was 30–0. I mention this not in a spirit of spitefulness, but just to show how unclear to the public can be issues which seem quite straightforward to the medical profession.

So it was in an uncertain frame of mind that I attended my first Colloquium—not the first that was convened, but the first to which I was invited. I gather that there had been some stormy disagreements at earlier sessions between the more intransigent parties on both sides. By the time I got there, the major fights had resolved themselves into something more like armed chess. At least the protagonists seemed to be playing the same game.

Men and women of good-will

What was the most striking at first sight was how similar the various practitioners seemed. Here were men and women who had trained exhaustively in their different disciplines, who had studied the body and its ailments, who had a pronounced view on how people react to various stimuli. Some were orthodox, some complementary. A sizeable number had had an orthodox training to which they had added an extra slant from some alternative form of medicine. On paper they might have seemed totally different. In the flesh, they came across as men and women of good-will working towards a common goal. This in itself was encouraging.

The big obstacle to any general agreement seemed, more and more, to be the theoretical bases of the therapies. It is just about impossible to believe all the alternative theories at once—if the acupuncturists' systems are correct, others can't be; the co-existence of allopathy and homoeopathy is a matter of continued wonder; to hear some (not all) osteopaths talk, you would think there was nothing that could not be cured by manipulation. Yet any one of the therapies can bring great benefit to some patients.

The way forward seemed to be to say "never mind for the moment *why* this heals; just consider if it *does*, and work backwards from there". The only thing which every form of therapy seemed to have in common was a reliance, greater or

138

less, on the springs of healing within the patient; an underground reservoir, if this is not being fanciful, that could be caused to gush forth by a very great variety of drilling equipment.

First, establish what happens

This is, properly considered, the very opposite of unscientific. Being scientific involves, as I understand it, first establishing what happens, and then trying to work out why. This is what all scientifically-minded people say they do, of course; but what people do, and say, can be very different things. Orwell knew this when he called the War Minister in his book "1984" the Minister for Peace, and the food rationing man the Minister of Plenty. Similarly, at Cambridge, there was a school of literary criticism which claimed only to dissect literature, paragraph by paragraph with no pre-conceived notions about the "greatness" of the authors. In practice, they had dogmas about what should and should not be read unrivalled since the Middle Ages.

In much the same way, in *theory* the more scientific you are, the more you look objectively at the evidence. In *practice*, the more you resist what you can't explain. Scientists are continually tempted to discount or ignore events for which no explanation is forthcoming. the most striking instance, I suppose, are meteorites, which for centuries proper scientists refused to investigate, since obviously only ignorant peasants would think that such big stones could fly through the air.

If we are to have a coming together of different therapies, therefore, we are going to have to stop arguing from our precepts of what ought to be, and look more and more at what actually *is*. This is the only method that can possibly encompass all the different therapies, and the most respectably scientific as well. And if it does turn out that in the vast majority of cases we are dealing with mechanisms which simply trigger the patient's own defences, then half the cause for fury and antagonism will have gone. It is not a coincidence that the BMA's somewhat scornful dismissal of all alternative therapies met with such an adverse public reaction, for it went contrary to the personal experience of too many people. And going against experience seems highly unscientific, whoever is doing it.

139

Three recollections

Now that the Colloquia are over, there are three things which stay in my mind particularly. The first, I was only able to read after the event, but it seemed to me to have enormous significance. This was Dr Patrick Pietroni's suggestion that the explanation of a great many things hitherto not understood might lie in the realm of the new physics. If there are forces other than those which have so far been studied, this would not only explain so much that is at the moment inexplicable—all the vagaries of psychosomatic medicine; the effects of "fringe" cures which seem to have no scientific base at the moment; the unsolved problem of why, exposed to the same risks and infections, some people get ill and some don't. It would also remove the major objection which scientifically-trained people have towards investigating such things. Ask a scientific man to run tests on some unexplained phenomena, and he cannot be blamed for refusing. Ask him to investigate a totally new branch of science, and even the most narrow minded can scarcely say no.

The second was a piece of historical anecdote retailed by Sir James Watt that Lister was indirectly involved in the tragedy of Captain Scott in the Antarctic. I have rarely heard a neater instance of how an excellent theory can become a disaster if it is applied too widely, nor that even in the most irreproachably "scientific" thinking there is far too much of fashion.

The third was, again, an anecdote, told by Professor Ian McColl. It concerned a family with a desperately sick child, who asked the doctor if he would mind if they took the child to Lourdes. Wishing no disrespect to the doctor's treatment, they nevertheless felt Lourdes might have something to offer. The doctor had the wisdom to say "Of course I don't mind; we need all the help we can get."

Seeking help from various sources

Easily the worst dilemma most of us face in our attitude to complementary practitioners is the extent to which recourse to them will undermine, alienate or enrage our own doctors, in whom we have certainly not ceased to trust. It seems a likely outcome of the advances made at the Colloquia that, increasingly, practitioners of different types will be able to see each others point of view, and the patient (who is, after all, the crux of the matter) will therefore be able to seek help wherever it seems possible to find it. I cannot think of an outcome of greater benefit, or more importance to us all.

Perspectives and Prospects

What has been achieved over a period of three years, as a result of these RSM Colloquia and other attempts at dialogue? Greater mutual respect between the orthodox and the complementary had led to complementary therapists being invited to join conventional medical care teams, and to the setting up of a number of joint research projects. Complementary practitioners have also taken a greater interest in rationalizing their own approach. The discussion has started to involve Government agencies and to be carried on at an international level. Undoubtedly, there will be a continuing dialogue into the Twenty-First Century

Perspectives and Prospects

Sir James Watt

Past President, Royal Society of Medicine

Since its inception, the Royal Society of Medicine has provided a forum for the debate of contemporary medical issues, many of a controversial nature. In the year 1842, at a meeting of its parent body, the Royal Medical and Chirurgical Society, a surgeon called W. S. Ward described how he had been able to carry out a painless amputation of the leg on a patient he had hypnotized by Mesmerism. His colleagues were sceptical. The patient was denounced as an imposter and all reference to the paper was deleted from the Society's minutes. That was because, as the scientist and philosopher, Sir Michael Polanyi has since observed, ''it is the normal practice of scientists to ignore evidence which appears incompatible with the accepted system of scientific knowledge.''[1] Today, the Royal Society of Medicine has a Section of Medical and Dental Hypnosis and its evidence enabled the BMA Working Party on Alternative Medicine to recommend the use of hypnotherapy by qualified doctors under certain conditions.

Professional self-interest
The story of 1842 is instructive, because it is still debatable whether or not hypnotherapy is susceptible to study by the scientific method, and it demonstrates the distrust between groups subscribing to different philosophical concepts which must be overcome in a spirit of honest inquiry if the contributions of each are to be effectively employed in the best interests of the patient. In his Fawley Foundation Lecture at the University of Southampton in 1967, Prince Philip observed that one of the less beneficial aspects of our changing environment had been the multiplication of specialist groups, which served narrow sectional interests to the detriment of the larger group—the nation state. Doctors were a case in point. Whereas they used to form an

145

important part of the local group with whom they worked, they had been forced to combine together in their own group. Group loyalty, however, led to conformity among those who would wish to be unconventional and, in an address to the Edinburgh Medical Group in 1971, Prince Philip appealed for a whole man and whole nation approach to health.[2]

The Colloquia, however, quickly demonstrated that professional self-interest was by no means confined to the medically qualified. The therapists were equally defensive and status-conscious and these attitudes were reflected in the differing perceptions, standards and goals which characterized their respective professional groups. The first major achievement of the Colloquia was to break down these barriers and, by demonstrating the professional competence of the therapists, to promote a favourable climate for the discussion of sensitive issues affecting the treatment of the patient as a whole.

Communication

This brought us to recognize the role of communication in relationships both with the patient and with professional colleagues. It was highlighted by a demonstration of the length and scope of the history taken by two therapists in contrast to the brief, limited encounter between a doctor and his patient, which, if commonplace, may account for some of the successful results of complementary therapies in the treatment of chronic or undifferentiated illness. Both conventional and complementary practitioners adopted a similar professional approach to history-taking, but the complementary practitioners enquired into a more exhaustive range of personal and environmental factors to reach a similar diagnosis.

Campbell has observed that failure of communication destroys personhood. But the converse is also true. The effort to communicate creates personal being, it invites response, creates new emotional bonds which replace prejudice by participation in the feelings of others and provides the basis for consistent and controlled interaction with them. Failure to communicate turns the other person into an inanimate object which can be manipulated in ways that suit us.[3] Any mechanical intrusion into this highly personal relationship, such as the use of

146

a computer for history taking, disrupts those very human interactions which may reveal psychological and spiritual needs for which appropriate counselling is required.

The problems of language

The Colloquia demonstrated, however, that communication between doctors and complementary practitioners ran into the same difficulty which often assails specialists and scientists attempting to collaborate with colleagues—the incomprehensibility of the language of the other's specialty. It became clear that, until the problem of language could be solved, doctors and therapists would continue to describe common concepts and phenomena in technical terms peculiar to their own specialty, which would perpetuate misunderstanding and generate mistrust.

Dr Patrick Pietroni has therefore rendered an invaluable service by describing the six languages currently used by doctors, research workers, health educators, psychiatrists and scientists to describe illness, some of whom even find impressive terms for non-existent illness. Fortunately, as he has shown, the problem is capable of resolution, as modern medical science moves away from rigid classical concepts to a general systems theory which embraces different systems of illness and explores their interaction in both biological and social terms.

It should therefore be possible for different concepts of illness to be reconciled through a common language, the terms which are intelligible to all responsible practitioners of the healing art.[4] The famous Eighteenth Century surgeon and scientist John Hunter would have approved of these developments. "Nothing in nature stands alone", he wrote; "every art and science has a relation to some other art or science: and it requires a knowledge of these others, as far as this connection takes place, to enable us to become perfect in that which engages our particular attention".[5] Recognition of the role of communication and language was therefore another important consequence of the Colloquia.

Discussion of changing scientific concepts enabled us to appreciate the effect of the infinite variety of influences upon the health of the cell and the implications of such factors as

147

environmental pollutants, food additives, home and working conditions, unemployment, personality, relationships, life-style and the media, for health and disease. If this called for a holistic approach to patient care, it also implied a team effort, by means of which many different skills: medical, scientific, technical, paramedical, complementary, pastoral and psychological, could be coordinated for the more effective support of patients.

Strength and weakness on both sides

The atmosphere generated by the Colloquia permitted both doctors and therapists to appraise their relative strengths and weaknesses. In his 1981 Reith Lectures, Professor Ian Kennedy criticized paternalistic attitudes and the cult of scientific medicine which gave doctors unlimited power to control the lives of others.[6] The Colloquia, however, revealed that most doctors were fully aware of the immense potential for benefit or harm of scientific medicine.

While welcoming the means it offered to cure or alleviate hitherto untreatable conditions, they nevertheless recognized its limitations in the management of chronic disease and the regretable consequences of over-prescribing, adverse drug reactions, inappropriate treatment and ultra-radical surgery arising from its emphasis upon survival and life-span rather than upon quality of living and ability to cope. Such consequences have caused some physicians to reappraise the significance of Twentieth Century therapeutic advances in view of the enormous cost of the biomedical research responsible for them.[7]

What they failed to recognize, however, was that it was unlikely that there would ever be enough time or money available to investigate fully those among the chronically unwell, for whom no diagnostic label can be found and the Colloquia left unanswered such important questions as: Who is to investigate them? What treatment do they require? Who is to give it? How is it to be done? Do they really need to see a doctor? Who decides and who does the initial screening?

The therapists, on the other hand, were often seen to be as much the prisoners of their own orthodoxy as the conventional defenders of Descartes. There was as much reluctance to admit paradox in their own philosophies as to acknowledge logic in

148

those of others and there was little evidence that any thought had been given to collaboration in joint therapeutic management. The therapists are private-practice orientated and it is to the credit of those professional bodies represented in the Colloquia that they were prepared to offer their skills for the benefit of National Health Service patients.

Public responsibility

Initial reluctance to validate some therapies changed throughout the Colloquia in the light of the public responsibility to prove efficacy. The Colloquia clearly demonstrated that those professional bodies which participated required high academic standards, several years of theoretical and practical training, a qualifying examination and the acceptance of a code of ethics, although it was considered that more clinical training was desirable in some therapies. In good hands their therapies were usually safe and they had good insights into their limitations and when to refer patients elsewhere. There was, therefore, no bar to collaboration with the medical profession. Unfortunately, the BMA Report did not distinguish between the qualified and the unqualified therapists.

In October 1986, before the conclusion of the Colloquia, *Which? Magazine* published a survey of members' attitudes to complementary medicine.[8] One in seven of its readers had visited a complementary therapist in 1985 and indeed regarded the treatment as complementary rather than as alternative to conventional medicine. Of these, 71% sought help because of pain or some musculo-skeletal condition; 15% had a psychological problem; 81% had sought advice from their GP and had been dissatisfied with conventional treatment; 82% claimed to have been improved or cured by complementary therapy; 14% found the treatment ineffective and 1% found that the problem became worse.* The point was made that conventional medicine treated the disease, whereas complementary therapists treated the person who had the disease and treatment was therefore tailored to individual needs. *Which?* considered that the BMA Report had shown the rift which existed

---

* This information is derived from data presented in schematic form in *Which? Magazine*.

between conventional and complementary Practitioners, and those most likely to suffer would be the patients. The report of the survey raised similar questions and proposed similar answers to those debated during the Colloquia.

Public protection

The protection of the public was a point made strongly by Baroness Trumpington and, throughout the Colloquia, the importance of comparable standards of training and qualification, a professional register and a coordinating body was repeatedly emphasized. The Council for Complementary and Alternative Medicine (CCAM) was formed in 1986, its founder members being the British Acupuncture Association and Register, the British Chiropractic Association, the British Naturopathic and Osteopathic Association, the College of Osteopaths, the National Institute of Medical Herbalists, the Register of Traditional Chinese Medicine, the Society of Homoeopaths and the Traditional Acupuncture Society. It has proved to be an active body which has already embarked upon a programme of self-validation in education and has examined the implications of registration.

Recognizing the need for research

The therapists have also recognized their public duty to show, if at all possible, how and why a particular treatment works, and an entire Colloquium was devoted to the consideration of research in this field. The BMA Working Party, for instance, was able to accept the role of acupuncture, osteopathy and chiropractic in pain relief, not because of well-documented clinical evidence, but because of the discovery, in a research laboratory in 1975, that the body's central nervous system produced its own analgesics, the endorphins. Subsequent study has suggested how these might be released by the use of acupuncture and the manipulative therapies.[9] Such serendipity is unlikely to be repeated and validation now will have to be sought through the design and use of an appropriate method.

Controlled clinical trials

The orthodox model, the randomized controlled clinical trial, is necessarily based upon groups selected for their strict comparability

150

according to strict entrance criteria which is fundamental beyond dispute. In view of the differing diagnostic criteria of conventional medicine and complementary therapy it does not appear possible to define a population which can be randomized for a controlled clinical trial of one form of therapy against another. It is because of difficulties with entrance criteria that physicians have recently turned to the use of randomized controlled trials in individual patients in order to identify the most beneficial treatment, and have reported some success.[10] It remains to be seen if this proves a useful model for the validation of the various therapies.

Research Council for Complementary Medicine

A significant development has been the advent of the Research Council for Complementary Medicine (RCCM) which contributed its President, Dr Richard Tonkin, and six Council members to the Colloquia Planning Group. It has exerted a most important influence upon the Colloquia, both directly and indirectly, by encouraging well-founded scientific research, by exploring methodologies which take account of individual idiosyncrasy, by exercising an enabling function for would-be researchers and, through its Scientific Information Centre, by providing research data in complementary medicine. One result of the Colloquium on Research was an invitation to complementary therapists, from hospital consultants associated with clinical research units, to learn research skills and participate in joint research projects. Regrettably, therapists have been rather slow to avail themselves of this opportunity and research in this field has been conducted mainly by medical personnel in university departments in collaboration with RCCM.

The British Holistic Medical Association

The contribution of RCCM to the Colloquia was paralleled by that of the British Holistic Medical Association (BHMA) which also encourages research, but concentrates upon the education of doctors, medical students and health care professionals in the principles and practice of holistic medicine. A recurrent theme during the Colloquia was the need to teach the medical profession, particularly those engaged in primary patient care, what complementary therapies have to offer, the principles

151

underlying their practice, the patients likely to benefit and the results to be anticipated. That such teaching is desirable stems from the increasing public interest in complementary therapies. Through its journal and seminars, BHMA is providing such essential information.

The Centre for Complementary Health Studies, University of Exeter

An important national development stemming from the Colloquia has been the founding of the Centre for Complementary Health Studies at the University of Exeter. The Centre will mount an integrated scientific exploration of complementary medicine by means of critical evaluation, research and seminars for doctors, those registered in the professions ancillary to medicine, and registered complementary practitioners; and there will be public lectures. It will also seek to establish recognized academic and legal standards. The Centre has now published a small but informative brochure on its activities.

The Institute for the Advancement of Health, New York

The Colloquia have also established an international dialogue. We have seen how other countries have examined the claims of complementary therapies and the role assigned to them within or outside the State health service. We have been shown patterns to follow and pitfalls to avoid and have ourselves contributed to the continuing debate. One important result of the Colloquia has been the liaison established between the Society and the Institute for the Advancement of Health in New York. This organization was founded in 1983 to further the scientific understanding of mind-body reactions in health and disease. It promotes research, encourages interdisciplinary exchange between scientists, clinicians and the health care professions and disseminates news of developments. Discussions have already been held on ways to collaborate.

Trends for the Twenty-First Century

The Colloquia revealed trends which may have implications for the practice of medicine in the Twenty-First Century. The chronic conditions of an aging population and illness resulting from environmental factors, tensions in society and the breakdown of family life, are likely to make disproportionate demands upon general practitioners to the detriment of patients more in need of their specifically medical skills. The escalating costs of high-technology medicine, competing for limited resources, will inevitably require a realistic review of priorities at a time when the demand for primary care is increasing.

The popularity of group activities, the response to challenge and the pursuit of physical fitness imply a more responsible public attitude towards both the community and personal health and well-being.[11] It explains the growth of fitness centres and the popularity of complementary therapy, which requires the active participation of the patient and emphasizes the body's natural capacity for self-healing. This appears to suggest that complementary therapists might find a future role in a community team of diverse therapeutic skills, thus relieving general practitioners of some of the burden and allowing them more time for the investigation and care of those patients whom they have been specifically trained to treat.

Multidisciplinary teams have already proved their worth, both in general practice and in hospitals. An imaginative research development is the Saint Marylebone Centre for Healing and Counselling in London, where a National Health practice, equipped with superb research facilities, has access to osteopathy, acupuncture, music therapy and Christian counselling all within this clinic.[12] Various members of that team made important contributions to the Colloquia, which provided evidence of growing interest, particularly among younger doctors, in complementary techniques and growing collaboration between medically qualified and non-medically qualified practitioners in other areas.[13] This, however, implies that changes are needed in medical education if such benefits are to be generally realized, and suggestions of how this ought to be achieved are contained in the body of the Report.

The Colloquia have nevertheless made it abundantly plain that the problem of provision of complementary therapies for the number of patients who are likely to require them cannot be solved by providing doctors with short-term or weekend courses

153

in a particular therapy; properly trained complementary therapists will be needed.

A catalyst for collaboration

By general consensus, the Colloquia succeeded in identifying problem areas in the practice both of orthodox scientific medicine and of alternative systems. They showed that a distinction exists between alternative practitioners who are in a position to offer a service complementary to medicine and those less able to do so. This distinction is mainly on the grounds of professional training, qualifications and codes of practice. The Colloquia indicated possible areas of collaboration between conventional and complementary practitioners and the steps to be taken to that end. They also acted as a catalyst in important collateral developments and it was agreed that the dialogue should continue.

Conclusions

In summary, the Colloquia:
1. identified some of the strengths and weaknesses of conventional medicine and complementary therapies;
2. distinguished between professionally trained and qualified practitioners offering a service to patients which is complementary to medicine and inadequately qualified therapists offering alternative systems;
3. noted the evidence of public demand for complementary therapy and discussed the safeguards required for public protection;
4. agreed that a whole-person approach may require changes in contemporary medical practice;
5. emphasized the importance of improved communication at all levels;
6. examined the problem of language and the need for the definition of terms;
7. noted some implications of advances in scientific concepts and the influence of environmental factors in health care;
8. highlighted the need for complementary practitioners to achieve recognized standards of training, to maintain a professional register and to establish a coordinating body.

This has since been realized in the formation of the Council for Complementary and Alternative Medicine;

9. endorsed the need for research validation of complementary therapies, recognized the difficulty in adopting orthodox research protocols to compare disparate therapies, welcomed the exploration of new research methodologies under the aegis of RCCM and the offers of research facilities from specialists in conventional disciplines;

10. noted areas such as chronic conditions and undifferentiated illness, in which complementary practitioners often have much to offer;

11. received accounts of the valuable contributions made by complementary therapists when participating in health-care teams both in hospital and in general practice;

12. emphasized the desirability for medical students and doctors to be better informed about complementary therapies;

13. initiated international dialogue;

14. acted as a catalyst in establishing the Centre for Complementary Health Studies at the University of Exeter;

15. examined the role which complementary therapists might play in the Twenty-First Century against a background of escalating health costs and a national trend towards personal responsibility for health, with the accent on self-help and on treatments designed to enhance the body's self-healing mechanisms;

16. recognized the importance of continuing the dialogue.

References

1 Polanyi M. *Personal Knowledge. Towards a Post-Critical Philosophy*. London: Routledge & Kegan Paul, 1973: 138.

2 HRH Prince Philip. Fawley Foundation Lecture, University of Southampton, 24 November 1967. Lecture on Health and the Environment to Edinburgh Medical Group, 17 December 1971.

3 Campbell A V. *Moral Dilemmas in Medicine*. Edinburgh: Churchill Livingstone, 1972: 135–6.

4 Pietroni P C. The meaning of illness — holism dissected. *Journal of the Royal Society of Medicine* 1987; **80**: 357–60.

5 Hunter J. Quoted by Lord Smith in his Hunterian Oration: The Hunters and the arts. *Annals of the Royal College of Surgeons of England* 1975; **5**: 3–18.

6 Kennedy I. *The Unmasking of Medicine*. London: George Allen & Unwin, 1981.

7 Beeson P B. Changes in medical therapy during the past half century. *Medicine* 1980; **59**: 79–85.
8 *Which? Magazine.* Magic or medicine? 1986 October; 443–5.
9 Clement-Jones V, McLoughlin L, Tomlin S, Besser G M, Rees L H, Wen H L. Increased beta-endorphin but not met-encephalin levels in human cerebro-spinal fluid after acupuncture for recurrent pain. *Lancet* 1980; **2**: 946–9.
10 Guyatt G, Sackett D, Taylor W, Chong J, Roberts R, Pugsley S. Determining optimal therapy — randomized trials in individual patients. *New England Journal of Medicine* 1986; **314**: 889–92.
11 Watt A. Community health initiatives and their relationship to general practice. *Journal of the Royal College of General Practitioners* 1986; **36**: 72–3.
12 Hamel-Cooke C K, Cope D H P. Not an alternative medicine in St Marylebone Parish Church. *British Medical Journal* 1983; **287**: 1934–6.
13 Wharton R, Lewith G. Complementary medicine and the General Practitioner. *British Medical Journal* 1986; **292**; 1498–1500.

Appendix
Members of the Colloquia Planning Group

Glin Bennet MD FRCS FRCPsych
Consultant Senior Lecturer, Department of Mental Health
University of Bristol

Graham Bennette MA MB BChir (Secretary and Coordinator)
Medical Services Secretary
Royal Society of Medicine

Ronald Davey MB BS MFHom AKC
Medical Director, Blackie Foundation Trust

Roger Hill MA MTAcS
Director, Centre for Complementary Health Studies
University of Exeter

John Horder CBE MA MD FRCP
Past President, Royal College of General Practitioners

Ian Hutchinson DC (USA)
Past President, British Chiropractors Association

The Rt Hon The Lord Kindersley DL
Chairman, Commonwealth Development Corporation

Barry Lambert DO MRO
Chairman, General Council and Register of Osteopaths

George Lewith MA MB B Chir MRCP MRCGP
Director, Centre for the Study of Alternative Therapies
Southampton

Simon Mills MA MNIMH
Chairman, Council for Complementary and Alternative Medicine

Roger Newman Turner ND DO BAc MBNOA FBAcA
Editor, *British Journal of Acupuncture*

Patrick Pietroni MRCGP MRCP DCH
Senior Lecturer in General Practice
St Mary's Hospital Medical School

Dr Richard Tonkin MD FRCP
President, Research Council for Complementary Medicine

Sir James Watt KBE MD MS FRCP FRCS (Chairman)
Past President, Royal Society of Medicine.

Index

159

160

complementary medicine *(continued)*
professionalism of practitioners 6
public demand 94
rapprochement with conventional
  medicine 57
rate of usage in UK 123
reasons for seeking 15
referral to 15
requirement to validate healing
  methods 5, 6
requirement for training 88
research projects 61
and science 30
in South Africa 107–12
survey of therapies 16
training 37, 52, 116
tribal medicine in South Africa
  121
in United States of America
  113–20
unusual claims 25
confidentiality in counselling 134
consumer protection 80–1, 90–1
consumerism 93–4
Consumers Association 94
consumers' views of complementary
  therapies 149
conventional medicine 2
approach to acupuncture 20
changes in profession 86
cooperation with complementary
  practitioners 85
failings 15, 28–9
governmental attitude 7
holism 28
models of illness 16–18
practitioners 138
rapprochement with complementary medicine 57
and science 30
training programmes 52
undergraduate curriculum 2
Conventional Medicine and Complementary Therapies, Colloquia
  on 4–8
cooperation
between disciplines 85–7, 140–1

with medical profession in
  Maryland 117
coronary disease prevention 86
Council for Complementary and
  Alternative Medicine 37
role of 87
self-validation programme 91,
  150
umbrella organization 91
counselling 127, 129–35
principles 131–2
self-determination 133
Cyriax 102, 104

data collection 68
defensive mechanisms 60
dentistry 87–8
Dentists Act 87
Department of Health and Social
  Security (DHSS) 92, 93
Descartes, R 1
diagnostic tools 44
dietary therapy 103
digitalis 71
disease 58–9
current bio-medical viewpoint 49
organic 1, 2
process 70
doctor
–patient relationship 3, 34
approach to peptic ulcer 17–18
collaboration with therapists 25
general practice and interest in
  complementary medicine 16
holistic approach 28
pastoral role 29
role of 1, 2
drug evaluation 67
Dutch Medical Association 99, 105
dying 2
quality of 31

ECG 44
education
in complementary therapies in
  South Africa 107
complementary therapy 89–90

161

education *(continued)*
 influence of Rudolph Steiner   101
 medical student   89–90
 in Netherlands   104
 professional standards   87
 programmes for complementary
  and conventional medicine
  52–3
 standards for complementary
  practitioners   73, 92
Einstein, A   49–50
Eisenberg, D   118
electrical system of body   115
Encounters with Chi   118
endorphins   124
energetic dysfunction   18
epidemiology
 clinical statistics   44
 statistics in   45
ethical constraints for therapeutic
 activity   57

faith healing   103
food allergist   17–18
freedom of choice for consumer
 80–1, 88, 90–1

garlic   69
General Council and Register of
 Osteopaths   90, 124
General Medical Council
 role of   87
 surveillance of complementary
  therapies   91
general practitioner
 and acupuncture   103
 and anthroposophical medicine
  101–2, 103–4
 and complementary therapists
  25
 diagnosis of illness   18
 and homoeopathy   101, 103
 information on complementary
  therapies   90
 manual therapy   104
 in Netherlands   100
 patients' changing needs   36

role as health broker   91
 training model for undifferentiated illness   19
Greer, C   114

Hamel-Cooke, Rev C   10, 33
Harvey, W   30
hay fever, trial of homoeopathic
 treatment   68
healing
 art of   1
 force of nature   59
 and science   34
 systems of   52–4
 value of intuitive knowledge   66
health   58–9
 care and competition in meeting
  demand   85
 costs of workers   115
 current bio-medical viewpoint   49
 primary care in South Africa   112
Health is for God   10
Heisenberg, W   50
heliotherapy   103
herbalism   102
 comprehensive systems of healing
  52
 isolation of practitioners   70
 medicines and the Medicines
  Act   73, 77
 remedies   73, 78–9
 representation at Colloquia on
  Conventional Medicine and
  Complementary Therapies   4
 research   67, 68–9
 in South Africa   109
 standards of practice   90
 in treatment of burns   125
 in United States of America   116
Hippocrates   59
holism   33
holistic
 approach   28, 75
 communication   3
 medicine   65, 151–2
homoeopaths
 Kentian   17

163

manipulative therapy
  acceptance in France 7
  by medical practitioners 86
  research 67, 68
  standards of practice 90
  manual therapy 102, 103
  in general practice 104
  training in Netherlands 104
Medical
  Act (1511) 89
  Aid Schemes in South Africa
    111
  Dental and Supplementary Health
    Services Professions Act (1974)
    109
  Research Council and attitude to
    complementary therapies 92
  Society of London 46
medical insurance funds 93, 94,
    103, 105
medicine in twenty-first century
    152–4
medicines
  proof of efficacy 78–9
  protection from unsafe and
    ineffective 76
  quality of manufacture 78
  safety 78
  unsubstantiated claims 79
Medicines Act
  (1971) 77–80
  special considerations for homoe-
    opathy 94
medico-legal problems 87, 93–4
mentally handicapped children 101
Mesmerism 145
mistakes, professional 137–8
Mitterand, President 7–8
mortality statistics 45
multidisciplinary teams 153
musculoskeletal medicine data
    bank 122

National Health Service
  benefits of integration of comp-
    lementary therapists 62–3
  budget 2

competing demands 2
and complementary medicine
    34, 92–3
funding 92
inclusion of osteopathy 88, 94
natural therapy 103
naturopathy
  biological energy in therapy 20
  representation at Colloquia on
    Conventional Medicine and
    Complementary Therapies 4
  in South Africa 109
Netherlands, medical laws 99
neuroendocrine pathways 28
Niehans, P 102
night cramps, homoeopathic control
    71
nurses, medico-legal problems 87

obstetric analgesia, homoeopathic
  control 71
occupational therapist 122
orthopaedic surgery 86, 115–16
osteopathy
  biological energy in therapy 20
  comprehensive systems of healing
    52
  in National Health Service 88,
    94
  in Netherlands 102
  referral for from doctors 87
  representation at Colloquia on
    Conventional Medicine and
    Complementary Therapies 4
  in South Africa 109
  training 95
  in United States of America 88,
    116

parenteral enzyme therapy 102
pastoralism 29, 129, 130
patent medicines 45
pathology, establishment of common
    86
patient
  –doctor relationship 3, 34
  –therapist interaction 60, 69

164

patient *(continued)*
  attitude 60
  and attitude of medical pract-
    itioners 23
  chronically unwell 148
  in clinical setting 15
  contact with pharmacists 89
  disruption of life by therapy 24
  examination 6
  factors in treatment 24
  freedom of choice 80–1, 88, 90–1
  history taking 6, 17
  holistic approach 36
  individual response 60
  involvement in investigation and
    research 67
  legislation and 34
  as a person 35–6
  protection 34, 90–1
  reasons for use of alternative
    medicine 82
  self-healing ability 3
  spiritual well-being 69
  state of mind 60
  subjective reactions to treatment
    68
Patient's Association 137
peptic ulcer, approaches of different
  disciplines 17–18
personality types and pathology
  67
pertussin, homoeopathic use 68
pharmacists
  patient contact 89
  in South Africa 111
pharmacology and homoeopathy
  20
philosophy of
  methods 86–7
  therapy 93
physical fitness 153
physicians, social status 45
physiology, correlation with traditional energetic concepts 67
physiotherapists and medico-legal
  problems 87
physiotherapy 102

phytotherapy 102
placebo
  in clinical trials 41
  effect 43, 60, 70
Plato 51–2
Plotinus 50–1
politics in medical profession 88
Popper, K 54
pre-pathology 67
preventive medicine 44
Prigogine, I 50
promotion of medical staff 53
psyche 28
psycho-therapeutic procedures 18
psychological pressures and effect on
  clinically measurable disease
  19
psychometric questionnaires, computerized 62
psychosocial
  factors in treatment 33
  therapy 70
public
  attitudes 10
  protection 150
  understanding of complementary
    therapists 33
  understanding of medical pro-
    fession 33
publication
  of guidance and advice on comp-
    lementary medicine 58
  of research 45, 53

radiation therapy and use of acupuncture for side effects 118
randomization 44
records
  keeping 68
  value of 71
registrars' research projects 61
regulatory mechanisms 60
reimbursement schemes 92
reparative mechanisms 60
research
  current approaches 66
  experiental technique 61

research (continued)
  funding 71-2
  involvement of complementary
    practitioners in clinical research
    71
  methodology 66-7
  methods for holistic perspectives
    67
  necessity for evaluation of comp-
    lementary medicine 57-8
  need for 150
  problems in complementary
    medicine 60-2
  projects by registrars 61
  protocols for complementary
    medicine 67
Research Council for Complementary
  Medicine 6, 61, 151
  design of research protocols 67
  links with universities 72
  survey of therapy 16
Royal Society of Medicine
  colloquia 4-8
  Section of Medical and Dental
    Hypnosis 145

Saint Marylebone Centre for Healing
  and Counselling 153
science
  and healing 34
  history of 30
  intellectual honesty 30
  and medicine 21
  and non-science 29-30
  in relation to cures 140
scientific method, appropriateness
  of therapy for human beings
  5
Scott, R F 126, 140
scurvy 125, 126
  planned trial 42
self-healing 3, 59
social workers 129, 130
soma 28
South African
  Department of Health 107
  Health Care Delivery System 112

spiritual healing 10
State Commission on Alternative
  Therapies (Netherlands) 100
statistics
  in clinical trials 41, 43, 44
  development of methods 46
Steiner, R 101
steroid responses in children with
  nephrotic syndrome 71
stethoscope 44
streptomycin, clinical trial 44
stress, positive 60
Supplementary Health Service
  Professions (South Africa) 107
surgeons, social status 45
surgery and therapeutic evaluation
  44
symptoms and organic disease 2

terminal illness 2
The Body Electric 115
The Emerging Field of Psychoneuroimmunology 62
The Experiences of South Africans
  relative to Chiropractic and
  Homoeopathy 108
therapeutic advances 148
therapeutic evaluation
  dogmatic 41
  empiric 41-2
  methods 65, 67
  research in 57
  in surgery 44
Third World medicine 36
touch, calming effects 68
training
  academic requirements in South
    Africa 121
  in complementary medicine 70
  in complementary medicine in
    South Africa 111
  standards for complementary
    practitioners 73
  in United States of America 117,
    119
treatment practice 86
tribal medicine in South Africa 121

166